Expecting

The Inner Life
of Pregnancy

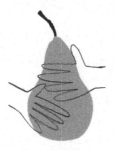

Chitra
Ramaswamy

Saraband

Published by Saraband
Suite 202, 98 Woodlands Road
Glasgow, G3 6HB, Scotland
www.saraband.net

ISBN: 9781910192214
ebook: 9781910192221

Printed in the EU on sustainably sourced paper.

10 9 8 7 6 5 4 3 2 1

For my son, the one I was expecting all along...

I'm a riddle in nine syllables,
An elephant, a ponderous house,
A melon strolling on two tendrils.
O red fruit, ivory, fine timbers!
This loaf's big with its yeasty rising.
Money's new-minted in this fat purse.
I'm a means, a stage, a cow in calf.
I've eaten a bag of green apples,
Boarded the train there's no getting off.
　　'Metaphors', Sylvia Plath

I'm a cloud, congealed around a central object, the shape of
a pear, which is hard and more real than I am and glows
red within its translucent wrapping. Inside it is a space,
huge as the sky at night and dark and curved like that,
though black-red rather than black. Pinpoints of light swell,
sparkle, burst and shrivel within it, countless as stars.
　　The Handmaid's Tale, Margaret Atwood

Send us, bright one, light one, Horhorn, quickening and
wombfruit. Hoopsa, boyaboy, hoopsa!
　　Ulysses, James Joyce

One

November

But the beginning of things, of a world especially, is necessarily vague, tangled, chaotic, and exceedingly disturbing. How few of us ever emerge from such beginning! How many souls perish in its tumult!

The Awakening, Kate Chopin

An unremarkable Sunday morning in November. A noir-ish time of year when nature's reel turns monochrome and the world becomes as smudged as old newsprint. Sombre November, as TS Eliot called it. The last gasps of another year. On the morning dog walk the leaves were pockmarked from an excess of autumn and had lost their florid complexion. They were beginning to blacken now and stick to my shoes as though slick with a thin layer of oil. It was the eleventh month of the year, though *Novem* means nine for it was the ninth month in the Roman calendar. Nine months. A clue dropped by a season, like so many leaves.

And so with all this promise of death I found myself taking a test proposing life. A frightening test, though perhaps there is no other kind. A test taken by oneself in the privacy of one's own bathroom towards the end of another year. A test whose result is revealed not by a mark on a page but by a stream of one's own bog-standard urine. A test for which there are only two results. Either life is there, burrowing in a place as close to you as your own heartbeat yet as mysterious as the inside of a mountain, or it is not and life, the other kind, goes on. How very simple. And how brutal too.

Expecting

Like however many millions of women before me and who knows how many in tandem, I squatted, hovered, took aim and waited for a blue cross to materialise in a tiny window of possibility. I had done this a few times in my life. In Glasgow in my early twenties when my partner at the time had just moved to London and I felt vengeful and very alone. The result? Relief. Or more recently in Soho, in one of the new breed of budget design hotels characterised by receptions without people and rooms without windows. That time? Disappointment. On both these occasions, the result had been negative. Life, the other kind, had gone on.

This time was different and as is often the case with major moments, I knew before I knew. I had eaten oysters twice in the previous week – unusual in itself and almost wilful in retrospect – and felt seasick as each sup slid down my throat. I had drunk whisky, smoked roll-ups and sung along to the Proclaimers in Edinburgh's The Port O' Leith, which in its own salty way is no less glamorous than sipping Bellinis in Venice or going for bagels in New York. The Porty, as it's known to locals, is an icon of Leith on my street, with its skew-whiff nautical decor and rousing nightly rendition of 'Sunshine on Leith' when last orders are called. But instead of feeling the euphoria that comes from belting out 'sorrrrroooowwww' with the bonfire of Laphroaig on my breath and the scent of the Firth of Forth on the air, I felt jittery. Five days previously, there had been a small rusty mark on a pair of pants, a question mark written in blood. It was enough of a hint for me.

And yet I had cause to doubt what is known in the business of trying to conceive – and one soon discovers that it is first and foremost a business – as an implantation bleed. That is, the moment when the ball of cells that goes by the dramatic name of a blastocyst burrows into the wall of the uterus, the most minuscule of plants taking root and making the ground shed tears of blood in response. Little blastocyst blasting its way into the world, so small and uncertain it has yet even to become embryonic.

My partner and I had been trying to make this everyday miracle happen for almost eighteen months. It had not been easy for us. We were two women for a start. The story was the kind of romantic comedy that would never get made, with all the madcap races across cities and highly charged encounters in hotel rooms you might expect. Stories that were good for dinner parties but bad for life. We had already done so much. Our preparation had been flawless; all we lacked was an outcome.

To start, a civil partnership to ensure we would both be the parents of a baby that might never be, a leap of faith that no heterosexual couple is required to make. Bizarrely, this needed to take place not just before birth but before conception, making the most private of acts a matter of public interest from the outset. And so it went on. Three donors and three corresponding excruciating encounters up and down the country. Home insemination kits bought off websites with deflating names like prideangel and fertilityzone. Blood tests at the GP's to ensure I was fertile. Dispiriting monthly trips to buy yet more ovulation tests, cruelly addictive (and expensive) little sticks that so resembled pregnancy tests I began to feel dumbly thrilled when they showed up positive. Then a growing obsession with donor profiles on international cryobank sites, where you can buy sperm by the syringe and have it delivered to you in a hissing nitrogen tank, which if nothing else sounds like the birth of a post-modern superhero. And finally, a number of exchanges in a series of hotels with neither windows nor souls.

Expecting

Every month, these brief encounters grew at once more workaday and strange. They began to gain an air of desperation, of waning passion and lost faith, sentiments that afflict most clandestine hotel trysts in the end. And the fact was they weren't working. Like November, we remained sombre, in limbo, aching for our lives to turn Technicolor, to end and begin again. The frustration that comes when your body refuses to submit to your will grew exponentially, fattening like the foetus it seemed would never be. Meanwhile, I grew increasingly defiant towards my own flesh and blood. I knew my body less and less with each passing month, just as we slowly grow to see a partner we no longer love as a stranger. To fail to get pregnant when one badly wants to is to engage in the most treacherous kind of battle: with one's own innards. We can no more will a baby into our bodies than we can draw an illness out of them.

Now I waited once more. Watched the beads of condensation on the cistern as they trembled, brimmed over and wept. Listened to the pigeon that had taken up residence outside our bathroom window for much of the autumn cooing with the persistence of a clock. Pictured Claire, my partner of eight years, a few feet away in the sitting room with the dog curled at her feet, waiting too. Witnessed the world distil itself, telescoped by anticipation into a chain of beautiful moments. Like words, life has a way of becoming poetry when slowed down.

You must wait three minutes before reading a pregnancy test. The length of a pop song or an ad break. During this time I found myself feigning nonchalance for the benefit of no one but myself, imagining a camera lens hovering above my head as we do when we sense something monumental is afoot. I left the bathroom, paced our hall, allowed myself a Hitchcockian moment of suspense with all its long shadows

4

and discordant strings, and then returned to the scene on which the plot of my life suddenly hinged. Finally I allowed myself a close-up. There it was. The revelation I had been imagining for so long. A moment not entirely unlike the adverts on television with their staunchly white couples flashing white teeth against white backgrounds, making fertility look oddly sterile, as innocent as ordering a salad for lunch. The vertical line was a little less significant than the horizontal, but it was a blue cross nonetheless. And beside it, an idiot's guide to deciphering the message. + = pregnant. - = not pregnant. A turning point, the kind that is mammoth enough to be experienced twice. First as raw moment, all heartbeat and terror. Second as story: dramatised, edited and reconstructed even as it unfolds.

'I'm a riddle in nine syllables,' wrote Sylvia Plath in her 1959 poem 'Metaphors'. Nine syllables. Nine lines. Nine months. The arc of pregnancy, with its triptych of trimesters, is as meticulously structured as a poem. Though, of course, one cannot break free of the conventions of pregnancy. There is no way to subvert its stanzas. Plath wrote these blackly humorous lines that peter out into quiet desperation when she was pregnant with her first child, Frieda. Six months after Frieda's birth on 1 April at home in London, Plath published her first collection of poetry, *The Colossus*. The birth of her baby marked her birth as a poet, but in many ways it was also the beginning of her death. Pregnancy symbolised Plath's own gestating consciousness, dark and wild, which she feared would consume her in the end. 'I have a fear, too, of bearing a deformed child,' she wrote years earlier in her journal of 1956, 'a cretin, growing dark and ugly in my belly, like that old corruption I always feared would break out from behind the bubbles of my eyes.'

Expecting

'Metaphors' is funny: the joke is on her, and on all pregnant women who are reduced to mere metaphors as they rise like yeasty loaves. Plath would remain as ambivalent towards motherhood as she was towards pregnancy for the rest of her short life. Or rather, she was a woman brave enough to spill its secrets, good and bad. And how could she have been otherwise at a time when the word itself was riddled with shame? When a pregnant woman was still a walking euphemism? In a family way. In a delicate condition. With child. Enceinte. Expecting.

Plath understood the tricksy nature of pregnancy, its deep and perplexing riddle, its silence as dark as the womb. She understood its peculiar contradiction: the problem of how you can be at your most lonely during the one time in your life when you are never alone. In philosophy the exploration of how a being relates to its world is known as the problem of self. Just think how this problem doubles, trebles, multiplies when there are at least two people inside one body. Plath understood what it was like to all of a sudden, after living with such unthinking ease in one's own body, feel like 'a means, a stage, a cow in calf'. She understood the wondrous absurdity of it. 'Vague as fog and looked for like mail. / Farther off than Australia,' she wrote in one of her most famous poems, 'You're', addressed to her unborn child. 'Right, like a well-done sum. / A clean slate, with your own face on.'

Plath made sense of pregnancy by travelling beyond experience to a place where only metaphor would do. Her approach was to write about pregnancy by not writing about it, by veiling it, perhaps even illuminating it, with metaphor. It was all too lonely a place to live in the end. In February 1963, while Frieda, then two, and her one-year-old brother Nicholas slept in their cots, Plath placed her head in the oven and turned on the gas. She put towels around the kitchen door so that the fumes would not reach her children. 'You are the one / Solid the spaces lean on, envious. / You are the baby in the barn,' she wrote in one of her last poems, 'Nick and the Candlestick', addressed to her baby boy. Her children had been her saviours. Yet Plath was imprisoned in the bell jar, an image that in its own way recalls pregnancy too. After all, pregnant women often feel trapped in their bodies, or rather their bodies become the trap. And isn't the womb, too, a kind of jar, albeit one we cannot look inside with the naked eye, one whose contents remain unseen until the lid is opened.

What, then, is the riddle of pregnancy? How are we even to begin to understand it? To find the right metaphors? Or perhaps even to abandon them: to crack open the jar and spill the contents? To cast aside the sentimentality, sanitisation, science, prescription, self-help, emotionally manipulative doggerel, lies, misconceptions, misogyny, unwanted advice, politicking, and the never-ending slew of news stories that serve only to patronise, petrify or pacify us? How do we find some meaningful understanding of one of the most thrilling, challenging and alien experiences of all? To describe what it really feels like to grow a person within a person? To tell the curiously silenced story of how every single one of us began?

Pregnancy. The word both sounded heavy in my mouth and suggested a kind of heaviness. It had something to do with its staccato rhythm, the way it began harshly and then finished with a soft purr, as if it were a pregnancy in reverse. It wasn't an easy word to speak aloud, just as it wasn't an easy experience to articulate. This made me like its awkwardness: it suited it. And what of its meaning? In Latin, *praegnans* translates literally as 'before birth'. It has long had a significance reaching beyond its description of the gestation of a foetus. There is the sense of pregnancy as carrying weight, depth or meaning. The pregnant pause. The pregnant moment. The pregnant utterance. By the late fourteenth century, to be pregnant also meant to be convincing, weighty or pithy. A pregnant argument was a compelling one. Then there was its sense of fullness and creativity. Its wonderful state of potentiality. I wanted to return to this definition of pregnancy as being ripe with meaning itself. To be pregnant with meaning as much as with child.

So much in pregnancy had been obscured by euphemism and it had happened over centuries. It was an experience that despite (or perhaps because of) being so unspeakable, has always been loaded with verbiage. The word 'pregnant' was itself a metaphor. Then there were all the historical synonyms – heavy, great-bellied, teeming, bound, pagled, bagged. And finally the sayings and expressions, varying across the world and ranging in tone and meaning from descriptive, humorous and prudish to derogatory and simply weird: up the pole (first used to denote pregnancy in *Ulysses*), bun in the oven (or, in French, 'bacon in the drawer'), knocked up, in pig, in the family way, stung by a serpent.

There was also the trajectory of the thing itself. In a time when haste and choice and control meant everything, a pregnancy could not be speeded up. It was a journey characterised by its length, stubbornness and difficulty, and an ascent that had to be undertaken all the way to its peak. There was no veering off course. The journey was laid out before me: charted by nature herself. Though mountaineering seemed the most masculine of sports – the need to conquer, to get to the top and survey the world from its ceiling – here was perhaps the most challenging climb that the body could make, and it was indisputably feminine. I wanted to chart my pregnancy as one might a great journey, follow it as one might a trail. Walk the river all the way back to its source. Find a new route to the summit of Everest. My body would become a map. No, it would become the landscape itself. Its contours would be the topography, each month would become a milestone, each trimester a landmark. I might tick off rare moments with the satisfaction of a birder. I might mark months with the relish of a hiker bagging Munros. I might even enjoy getting lost. And what of birth? It would become the resting place. The end of the line. The top of the mountain. The final destination. The place where the wild things are. 'The black force,' as Plath called it in her extraordinarily detailed description of Nicholas's birth, also at home, in her 1962 journal. 'I had nothing to do with it. It controlled me.' And then? The product, the issue, the baby in the barn.

Later that day Claire and I went for a walk in the Hermitage, an ancient woodland straight out of a Grimm's fairytale and the kind of sheltered place that is particularly prized in a northern city blasted by wind and haar. The kind you burrow into, which seemed apt for that other journey on which I was embarking. In fact, this twelfth-century former hunting ground would bookend my pregnancy. Exactly forty-two weeks later I would wind up back in this deep green gorge, beating the very same paths on the day I went into labour.

Even in Edinburgh, where a daily commute through a medieval town carved into ice-age rock makes you somewhat inured to all things old, the Hermitage feels ancient. These are surely the oldest trees in the city, as gnarled and characterful as storybook giants. Ash, beech, sycamore. Weathered, wide, Victorian in age and grandeur. Though wild boar and deer were once hunted here, these days you're more likely to see locals in Hunter wellies calling on their Labradors, who invariably go by the name of Monty. As usual Claire and I made for an unusual couple, a sentiment so familiar it perversely made me more at home. Like all happy outsiders, I have always felt most myself in the places where I fit in the least. Well, here we were: two women, one Anglo-Indian, one Scottish, walking that most maligned and working class of dogs, the Staffordshire cross. And something else accompanying us too, a secret, a potentiality. Whenever fellow dog walkers asked a question about our dog, only one of us would be addressed, as though it were unfathomable for both of us to own her. If this was the case with a dog, how would we be seen – or rather not seen – with a baby?

We wandered in a daze, barely talking. I felt that odd commingling of excitement and dread that comes with getting what you want. My belly, as flat and featureless as a field, whirled with wish-fulfilment and a sense of the unknown as our dog thundered up the slopes ahead of us in search of squirrels. Everything as it always was, everything utterly changed. I felt too jumpy even to place a hand on my own stomach, which suddenly seemed to belong to someone else. Despite my long-held belief that a woman's rights override those of her foetus, I felt that perhaps it did.

Our news was still new, as unspoken and frightening as a family secret. We were shocked by it, and this too was shocking, for how can something you've been planning so meticulously still surprise you when it comes off? The fact is I had been trying to conceive for so long that I had forgotten the point of it all. I was like the fisherman so stunned by the catch squirming on the end of his line that he throws it back in the water. The ritual of the rod, the river and the lure had so consumed me I had forgotten about the fish. And now that I had come to the end of the line, I realised that, like so many ends, it was only another beginning. This, too, was part of pregnancy's riddle.

The following morning, just to be sure, I did another test. Another blue cross. Another aftershock, smaller but still seismic. These two tests were my gathering evidence and were infinitely more convincing than anything that was happening inside my body, which seemed like an abstraction next to something so concrete, so external. That pale blue cross meant so much more to me than what was taking place inside a body I no longer knew. I carried those two sticks around for weeks, feared them like a superstitious person fears a rabbit's foot, for any object imbued with such power resonates with both good and bad luck. Meanwhile I felt nothing. My body remained a stranger. I didn't feel pregnant, but I did feel altered, like a walking phantom limb. No, even more transported than that. It was as though I had switched places with my shadow and was destined now to follow my body at a slant, disappearing here and lengthening there, climbing up walls or rippling over pavements, lagging behind or jumping ahead. I felt furtive like a shadow, too. Slippery.

A week later I was at the Early Pregnancy Unit, awaiting my first scan. It is not customary to have a scan before twelve weeks but there was some concern I might have an ectopic pregnancy, one in which the fertilised egg implants outside the uterus. There had been a little spotting but I was oddly unperturbed. I am not given to such boundless optimism but I was already realising something unexpected about my expecting self. Her responses were slower, not in a lumbering, mindless way, but slow like the tortoise who wins the race. I would need to get to know this creature, just as I would need to get to know the one slowing her down.

Expecting

As well as all the staid, enduring, Athens-of-the-North stuff, Edinburgh is a city of surgeons. Doctors from all over the world have for centuries been drawn to this small capital hemmed in by the sea on one side and an extinct volcano on the other. It has a medical feel to it that is difficult to place: one gets the sense that a lot of ancient body parts in formaldehyde lurk behind the doors of its elegant buildings. Newness sticks out in what Muriel Spark called 'the city of Calvinism, high teas and loveless alliances', destined always to feel like a flash in the pan.

The Early Pregnancy Unit is at the Royal Infirmary, a particularly brutish example of the new and home to Scotland's biggest maternity unit. More than six thousand babies are born here every year. As Claire and I arrived I recalled my father, one of those men with a great respect for medicine until it's being applied to himself, on his first visit to the city. He lifted his large nose, the same one I inherited at birth, and took in a long, theatrical draw of Edinburgh's particular brew of hops and cold sea air. 'Hmmmm,' he said, with a reluctant sense of awe. 'Smells like solicitors and surgeons.'

In keeping with all this, the hospital has a long and illustrious history of delivering babies. It was here in Edinburgh, in 1847, that James Simpson became the world's first doctor to use ether and later chloroform in a case of childbirth. For this desire to relieve the suffering of women he was condemned, both by the establishment and the clergy who accused him of 'seeking to rob God of the cries of anguish and the pleas for forgiveness which sinful women require to express during childbirth'. In 1872, two years after Simpson's funeral, the largest the capital had ever seen, the Edinburgh Royal Maternity Hospital – the first dedicated unit of its kind in the city – opened as part of what was described as 'probably the best planned hospital' in Britain. By 1939, almost a decade before the establishment of the National Health Service, the Simpson Memorial Maternity Pavilion had opened next to the main Victorian hospital. It must have been a great source of pride. Indeed, entire generations of Edinburghers, including much of Claire's family, continue to fondly refer to themselves and their own as Simpson's babies.

These days it's a different story, one of the NHS in microcosm. The original Victorian building is now part of the Quartermile development, a joint venture by a bank and 'conglomerate' that houses converted luxury apartments, offices, newbuilds, artisan bakeries, mini-supermarkets and various other aspirations that tend to come with so much glass and stone. The new £190-million purpose-built Royal Infirmary, funded by private finance, is far away on the southern outskirts of the city and must be reached by car or a long, gloomy journey on a bus mostly populated by pensioners travelling solo. The majority of the site, which opened in 2003, feels as if it's taken up with a sprawl of alphabetised car parks. Charges apply, of course.

Anyone who has had the misfortune of going to hospital this century knows the drill. The walk past the huddle of inpatients who may or may not be auditioning for a Beckett play, smoking outside the entrances in dressing gowns. The revolving doors emblazoned with the inflammatory words: 'One in three of us has bacteria that can kill!' Once inside, the shops, providing that ever-present retail hum, which is reassuring at first and then sinister when you remember why you are here. WHSmith, a bank, hairdresser, clothes shop and café selling packet sandwiches and bad coffee. The branding everywhere, a constant reminder that you have entered the age of the hospital as corporation, where patients are consumers and money buys life. The sound of your shoes squeaking over shined floors, as frightening as the boy riding his bike through the corridors of the Overlook Hotel in *The Shining*. The random patients lying on gurneys along the way, glassy-eyed, resigned, waiting. The feel of an airport lounge, of being manoeuvred this way and that, and the child-like resignation that comes with being told precisely where to go. Except the destinations here are places you hope you will never visit in your waking life. Neurosurgery, dialysis, palliative care.

When we arrived at our destination we sat beside two other sets of couples, avoiding eye contact as is customary in any British waiting room where there is a common purpose. I had been told not to go to the toilet as a full bladder makes for a clearer scan. And so we all sat sipping water and crossing and uncrossing our legs with the choreographed rhythm of characters in a BBC comedy sketch. My eyes were drawn to a poster – a warning about something or other – of a woman's distended belly in close-up. A bump, as it is known in the oddly disembodied language of pregnancy. The most rotund of tundras. Her belly button, once a deep pool, had flattened into a crater on an arc of pale moon. There was a vertical, not-quite-straight line running from rib cage to pubis. A ley line across an open field. And in the midst of this awesome bodyscape a hand, tiny and perfectly formed, reaching out through skin. A starfish drifted up from the bottom of the sea. A disturbance at the earth's core. I reacted to that poster like a healthy person reacts to illness. It seemed impossible; like something that could happen only to someone else.

Inside the examination room the routine began. Some blood was taken from my arm to test how much of the pregnancy hormone hCG, the one that produced those two blue crosses, was present in my body. A hell of a lot, which was why I was starting to feel sick. This is the hormone that creates the cells that make a placenta, the great bloody sea sponge that feeds a foetus for nine months. I lay down and a cool, clear jelly was applied to my stomach by a woman with an inscrutable face. She moved a small device called a transducer around like a gold-panner searching for treasure, homing in on particular areas and pressing down harder than I expected. She looked not at me, but at the monitor to her left. The room, like her face, was lit by its screen. This, combined with the drama of it all, made it feel like we were in a cinema. Claire and I even held hands in the dark like sweethearts on a first date. I held my breath and experienced the same delicious anticipation that comes when waiting for a movie to begin, the same delicious shyness felt when touching someone in the dark without looking at them.

There was no film to be seen. It was too early in the pregnancy and also I was told I had a tilted uterus. This would prove to be a characteristic experience of pregnancy: finding out bewildering facts about the body I thought I knew so well, usually divulged in such a mundane way that I wouldn't even think to ask what any of it meant. It was like opening my back door and discovering a whole new world in my garden. A tilted uterus. Claire asked if it would prove a problem during labour. That she was thinking so far ahead, already, shocked and touched me in equal measure. The answer was no. A tilted uterus was just as normal and healthy as one that didn't tilt. I listened to this short discussion about my womb with complete detachment. I had no idea what they were talking about.

The sonographer asked if I would consider an internal scan. I agreed, and removed my underwear, put my feet together, and dropped my knees. What felt like a speculum was inserted inside my vagina and up against my cervix, a tightening sensation familiar from years of smear tests, and the next thing I knew my uterus was on the monitor, a pulsing, shifting sea of

15

grey and foamy white. It was the most perfect thing. It looked so much like every other uterus in the world that it was hard to believe it was mine. This was my first view inside myself, yet I found it hard to grasp that it was my view, and it was of me. It reminded me of the first time I went to New York. Approaching the city from JFK, a tin can of an airport, in the requisite yellow cab driven by the requisite talky New Yorker, the famous skyline came into view. Steps in the air made of skyscrapers. *New York, New York. Taxi Driver. Breakfast at Tiffany's. Sex and the City.* I saw the things I couldn't see – a bridge over water, the Statue of Liberty punching the air, steam rising from drains, doormen blowing on their fingers outside Art Deco apartment blocks. The view was too iconic, too familiar, too obscured by its own image. It was superimposed on itself. I couldn't see it with my own eyes. I couldn't own this most famous of cityscapes for myself.

The same thing happened in that darkened room, looking at my own uterus. It was too iconic. Too womb-like. Too much its own metaphor. The more I saw, the less I saw. But there was more. In the upper left corner, if you could call it a corner, a tiny oval with a dot in the middle. A cartoon fried egg. An eye. The tiniest of black holes. It needed a professional eye to be seen, but once pointed out it was undeniable. My own little Big Bang. The beginning of it all.

We were sent back out to the everyday world of car parks and bodies you can't see inside with a scrap of paper. It looked like a handwritten receipt, the kind you get when you buy a piece of secondhand furniture. And just like a receipt, it was immediately lost in the nether regions of my bag, never to be seen again. But I remember exactly what it said. Pregnancy sac. 5–6 weeks. 6mm long. Three lines of terse, exquisite poetry. And not a metaphor in sight.

Two

December

O for God's sake
they are connected
underneath
    'Islands', Muriel Rukeyser

Our boat idled on neatly clipped waves, rising and falling like an animal breathing in her sleep. As close as you could get to stillness at sea. We had been gliding over the Indian Ocean for less than fifteen minutes but already there was no land in sight in any direction, just ever more water hugging the earth's curve all the way to the horizon. The most undiscovered part of the southern Maldives, just 50km from the equator. A middle-earth place with an end-of-the-world feel. A place where land is a mere interruption in water. Where islands this small and low-lying seem miraculous, nibbled yet somehow never swallowed by an insatiable sea. Not yet anyway. Where buildings, hospitals, car parks and scans seemed unimaginable. Where most of what's going on happens out of sight, beneath the water's skin, just as it is with the body in early pregnancy. I imagined the foetus sloshing around in my watery womb, a sea creature swimming in time with the boat creaking upon the wrinkled sea. I was living life in tandem now too. My secret had flown across the globe with me.

We were in one of the deepest and largest atolls in the world, its reefs untouched not only in the sensational language of travel guides but in the proper sense that no human hand had touched them. At least we had been assured of this by the manager of our island resort, an elegantly besuited anomaly in this elemental world. He said it with great pride, as though he had seen to the matter himself, when in actual fact his brand new hotel arranged along a curved kilometre of white sand was destroying the same ideal of remoteness it promised day by day. Here we were, after all, come to look but not touch. Here were the honeymooners and the young Indian families and the Chinese holidaymakers from supersized cities come to kick off their shoes and sink tired, too-long-encased feet in the sand. Everything in this warm shifting world was opposed to my own hard and sure land, which at that time was taken over by Christmas shoppers, the pavements slippery with frost first thing and soupy with grit by midday. Yet even here, thousands of miles away, I was pregnant. Somehow this was surprising, like the child's realisation that it is the same sun and moon that follow you wherever you go.

We set about the pleasing ritual of snorkelling; trying flippers for size and catching snorkels tossed to us by nimble Maldivian guides. Slender boys who rested their bare arms over the side of the boat like drivers do out of car windows on longed-for warm afternoons back home. These young men were as comfortable on water as I was on land. It was a pleasure to watch them at work, as it always is to see people doing what they do with skill and good grace. They busied themselves pointing at sights I could not see hidden in the scalloped waves. Gazed openly at a sky I could not look at it without sunglasses. All the time, the men, the water, what might lie beneath it, the sky, everything I saw, smelled, touched and thought was coloured with my ever-breaking news, the tiny bombshell I could throw overboard at any moment and watch as the circles printed the ocean like marks on a page – *I am pregnant.*

I loved the sea with a kind of defiance. I had learned to swim in my local pool beside a perilous dual carriageway near where I grew up in south-west London. On either side of this roaring road stretched a sixteenth-century former hunting ground called Old Deer Park. The swimming baths sat in the middle of the park, but it was the arterial road – its squall, size and the ominous bunches of flowers and little notes tied to trees along the route – that I remember most. You had to cross a brutalist bridge to get there and after a swim I loved to stand in the middle of it, arms dangling over, watching the cars zoom beneath me. The vibration of each one screaming up through my feet. The chlorine in my damp hair.

Years later I taught myself front crawl in Glasgow by reading a book about it that my boyfriend at the time borrowed from the library. We learned together, critiquing each other's strokes and racing one another up the length of the university pool. Perhaps swimming held a particular power for me because my parents hailed from a landlocked part of the world: a city on a plateau in the middle of the lower middle of India. The first sea they saw was probably Blackpool in the Eighties, and that was a memory of encountering racism, not water. Neither of them could swim. I had found this embarrassing as a child, unable to understand it as a result of their immigrant experience. Or perhaps I did understand, but it only shamed me more.

A childhood beach holiday somewhere in Spain. Costa del Sol. A walk through a dry, fragrant pine forest until the carpet of needles and dropped cones underfoot mingled with sand. First view of the Mediterranean Sea, a calm blue line shimmering over yolk-yellow sand. The oddity of seeing my mother and father, always in sari and suit, in clothes I associated with white people: swimming costume and trunks. How it frightened me a little. Holding my mother's hand in the shallows and feeling the surf fizz around my skinny thighs. The thrill of cold water slapping my tummy. Then panic. A modest wave hit and my mother fell and went under. The water must only have gone up to her ankles yet somehow I remember it closing over her head. The terror of seeing the rock in my life submerged. Trying to cling to her slippery hand as it flapped this way and that like a fish on a deck. Feeling the terrifying responsibility of the child momentarily forced into adult. Then she raised herself up and it was all over. We staggered out of the sea, I was wrapped in the swirly Seventies towel that seemed to accompany us everywhere, placed upon a stripy deckchair to kick the sand off my feet, and that was that. How different it would be for the third generation inside me. How we would swim together.

I spat into my mask, attached it to my face with a satisfying snap, and bit down on the warm plastic of my snorkel. Then came the shuffle to the edge of the boat, the chivalrous hand down from one of the young men that always makes one feel oafish and middle aged, and the plunge into cool water. The frightening awareness of a whole other world swaying beneath my kicking legs, the place where all life on our planet began, and the chilling view of oneself corrupted by too many viewings of *Jaws*. Legs more pale and child-like when peered at underwater. The sense of space tunnelling down and down like a vertical view of a mountain range. Then eventually darkness. Silence. Pressure. Weird sea creatures lit like jukeboxes. The earth's womb.

I dipped my head under and looked around in a frenzy,

desperate to take in everything at once in the same way one consumes the last few pages of a book too fast. Schools of sweetlips, angelfish, parrotfish, clownfish, too many fish to count or name. Cities of coral, nature's architecture, in every palate and design. And then, once I had adjusted to this knobbled metropolis, a turtle ambling along the edge of the reef before spinning off into the deep and disappearing. Rays like silk handkerchiefs, slipping over one another with the rhythm of synchronised swimmers. And most remarkable of all, a lone white-tipped reef shark slicing through the water directly below my stomach. Below my own little goldfish bowl. It was too soon and yet I couldn't help it. I found myself speaking to the thing inside me. It was roughly the size and shape of a tadpole, curved and sightless, a creature more suited to this world than the one in which I lived and breathed.

'Look!' I whispered. 'A shark!' And with this encounter came a realisation: I was no longer by myself. Not even here, under the sea, a lone swimmer crossing paths with a lone shark.

I had almost cancelled this trip. I was here for work, a press trip, or what journalists with varying levels of embarrassment like to call a perk of the job. Early pregnancy feels fraught with danger even when you're sitting on your own sofa. The risk of miscarriage is higher in the first twelve weeks. Things can and do go wrong for all sorts of mysterious reasons and this gives you a constant feeling of wariness, that nervy sense of 'why tempt fate?'. Also, you're on your own, sealed in by secrecy. The threat of miscarriage dictates that you keep the news to yourself for twelve weeks in case the worst happens. I followed this rule obediently without once questioning it. Just like that, because society told me to, I told almost no one, moved gingerly, stroked my stomach, whispered to it beneath the waves, and hoped.

Expecting

The embryo was so small and yet it already demanded so much from me. I felt like a beehive: so much going on, so little to see. It was a time of staying in, feeling exhausted, and telling inane lies as to why you're not drinking alcohol. And yet here I was, thousands of miles from home, treading water in the middle of the ocean. The journey had been epic, taking almost twenty-four hours: two long-haul flights, a sea plane, a speedboat ride across rough seas. What would it feel like to miscarry on a speck of land in the middle of the Indian Ocean? What was I doing here?

I think I wanted to remain myself for as long as I could. To continue to be the kind of untethered person who could pack a bag, get on a plane and lower myself into an ocean on the other side of the world. I wasn't ready to give up on that yet. In fact, I wanted it more than ever: map of dried salt on my skin, horizons cutting the world in half, all the stuff you crave when your world shrinks to the view from your own window. There was a nine-month countdown on everything now. I was a walking egg timer who would eventually become Plath's absurd 'melon strolling on two tendrils'. I understood that this would be my last trip somewhere like this by myself for a very long time and this sobering knowledge had brought me here.

What I hadn't realised was that I wasn't by myself at all. And what was this thing residing in me? It seemed more fish than human. Didn't we begin, after all, as organisms drifting in the sea? Didn't we swim before we stood up and walked across the African plains? And here I was thinking about beginnings and the embryo was already one step ahead of me. It had graduated to a foetus, a Latin word for offspring. I liked the dynamism of that word, the way it suggested something springing off into the world. Little go-getter, determined to make it. Other things were happening too. It had a bump for a brain, a bulge for a heart, buds for limbs, and dimples for ears. Its hands were paddles, the tiniest of oars. Its skin was transparent, like an octopus revealing her ink. The nervous system was already beginning to take shape, the brain growing fast, cartilage forming.

As for me, my uterus had swollen to the size of a lemon but it felt more like a nut: small, hard and encased. I found myself trying to suck it in as one inevitably does in a bikini, and failing. It could not be breathed away. It felt heated, spicy almost, as though I had eaten chillies. I felt very inwardly active, like a volcano that had lain dormant for decades and was now awakening. I felt protective of my stomach too, squeamish even about pulling a seatbelt over it on the plane. Then there was my desire to nest. I loathed that word for all its connotations of Fifties housewives feeling compelled by nature to take up their feather dusters, and yet, here I was feeling it sharply and rudely in the twenty-first century. I wanted to make a nest and curl up in it. I wanted to be a nest.

That night we had dinner with the urbane manager on the beach, under the stars, feet in cool sand. We were a small, unlikely group. A sporty young woman from an airline magazine who had dived the best sites in the world and was convinced this atoll couldn't compete with Indonesia, a middle-aged woman who had won a travel-writing competition in a national newspaper and decided to jack in her job to become a full-time writer, and our publicist, a bright-eyed London girl with a different sarong to go with each bikini. None of them had children. Only one, the publicist, knew my secret. And then there was me, an in-between person in all senses: in between their ages and stages of life, in between loving men and women, in between not having and having children. I had never felt so unmoored.

At first we spoke carefully, batting back and forth well-worn travel stories and asking the manager the right questions about the resort. Eventually the conversation became more frank and we discussed the local heroin problem, the rumoured sightings of pirates, and the problem of trying to turn your average uninhabited, rat-, snake- and spider-infested island into paradise. That is, paradise as we Westerners would have it: the raked white sands, artfully placed palm trees, water villas with plunge pools and noiseless air conditioning and, above all, no creepy-crawlies. The resort was new and thus was still being sprayed daily with insect repellant, the very air we breathed sanitised like an aeroplane cabin before takeoff. We were warned that some mosquitos still remained and it would be best to sleep with our villa doors closed.

So a real island was just a piece of land that happened to be above water at this moment in time. True remoteness, one would want to escape rather than discover. We wanted the fantasy. We wanted our wildness as cultivated and orderly as a botanical garden. There were no untouched places after all, at least none on dry land, and it struck me, under that clear, cleansed night sky, that it was the same with pregnancy. The image of the beatific woman with milk-swollen breasts and baby-swollen bump was just that. An image as airbrushed and iconoclastic as Demi Moore on the cover of *Vanity Fair*. As beatified as Botticelli's Venus emerging from the shell, one hand hiding her pudendum in shame. The reality was so much more difficult than that and so much more hidden. You had to dive deep to find it. You had to be careful coming back up for air. You had to circle slowly or you might get the bends.

We left our crescent of sand in the early hours of the morning to begin the long journey home. There had been a storm brewing as I'd gone to bed the night before and I'd fallen asleep to the resounding smash of the ocean pounding the house reef over and over again. It was a noise that might have lulled me to sleep or at least excited me if I hadn't been pregnant, but that night it had frightened me. I'd thought of the nearest piece of land facing my little villa – Indonesia, 2,675km away over surging black ocean. When I rose a few hours later I felt sick and dizzy and the storm was in full force. The speedboat bucked in the churning sea as we staggered onboard from the jetty. I gripped onto its cool white side as we climbed enormous waves in a starless, soupy darkness, falling back to the water's surface with a horrifying smack. Up and down, over and over again. I tried to think, see and feel nothing. I could not dispel the pure and physical fear that seized my body, my heart and, I feared, my womb. Little helpless tadpole, fired from one side to the other. One of the Maldivian boys pulled me to the bow of the boat where the drop was less sheer. I clutched my stomach in terror and guilt, convinced I was about to be thrown overboard, that the foetus would die of fright, I would miscarry right there on the slippery floor of the boat as it soared and dropped and my red blood ran into white sea spray. Fifteen minutes later the roughest crossing I'd ever experienced was over and we were hauled, soaking and shaking, onto dry land. I felt stupid, reckless and grateful to have made it through what one of the boys referred to with a shrug as a completely normal crossing in a storm.

Back home, the sickness grew with each passing day. I woke up reeling with it and it ebbed and flowed through the day, like motion sickness – but the thing in motion was me.

Expecting

A peculiar taste in the mouth, smooth and slightly metallic like a conker pressed to the tongue. It was a shimmering nausea, heated, rich and thirst-inducing, that threatened but never quite delivered an actual purge. There was more to it, even, than plain old sickness. I felt attuned to things, like when you fall in love and the world arrests you all over again. The smell of a man's neck made me dizzy with its mingling of scratchy wool, aftershave and dry winter skin. The taste of December in my throat: woodsmoke, snow, after-work drinks. It was like acquiring a sixth sense. No, a kind of synaesthesia. I could sniff out the oily blackness of the wynds in Edinburgh where homeless men peed at night before I walked past them. Touch the pink-rimmed hangover of the person sitting next to me on the bus.

'It is in moments of illness that we are compelled to recognise that we live not alone,' wrote Marcel Proust, referring not to our kinship with others in pain, but with ourselves. '[We are] chained to a creature of a different kingdom, whole worlds apart, who has no knowledge of us and by whom it is impossible to make ourselves understood: our body.' Proust wasn't talking about pregnancy, obviously, but this alienation from the body hits doubly hard when one is also carrying an alien. Not only are we alienated by illness; we are also growing aliens.

Morning sickness was the illness with the false name that could strike morning, noon or night and affected more than half of all pregnant women, particularly in the first trimester. It was caused by an increase in levels of progesterone, the hormone that relaxes the muscles of the uterus and prevents early childbirth. That was one theory anyway. Another more powerful one did away with the pathology of it and explained this heightened level of perception in terms of evolution.

Two • December

Morning sickness was a way of protecting the foetus from toxins, which is why it mostly struck in those crucial first twelve weeks when it is most vulnerable. So perhaps the very sights and scents that were making my stomach turn – a blue-veined slab of beef and the damp stain it left on a wooden chopping board, a puddle of raw egg swilling in a bowl – were the ones to avoid. I liked this explanation. It made me feel like an animal sniffing her way through the world.

In truth I felt more ill than pregnant. The foetus was like a parasite, a lump, a growth drawing everything lively and good from me. I was too tired and sickly even to resent it. In the nineteenth century, one of the slang terms for pregnant was 'poisoned', a reference to the swelling involved and perhaps the sense that like a poison, the baby eventually needed drawing out. I understood this. After all, its strengthening spelled my weakening: it had to be so. I felt the topsy-turviness of it all keenly: the more ill I felt, the more healthy I was. Others agreed. When I told health professionals I was feeling sick, the response, invariably, was 'Great!'. Sickness was indeed a sign of good health. This was nature's perversity. To feel dreadful meant my hormones were growing at a monstrous rate, that the foetus was taking what it needed from me. So if there was illness to be borne, it was to be celebrated. Nurtured rather than treated.

And yet, how could something the size of a mere kidney bean be wreaking such havoc? There was almost no weight to it, it took up virtually no space in the world, yet it was a burden – and a secret one at that. There was enough of it to make me pee constantly, catch my breath at the top of a flight of stairs, and fall asleep in the early hours of the evening on the sofa. This young bean was turning me into an old woman. It filled my mouth with saliva and left me feeling excited, frightened and estranged from my own body. I had lived in this house of flesh and blood for years and now all of a sudden I knew nothing about it. How was it doing what it was doing without my understanding? How had I gone so long, knowing so little? For the first time ever, I thought I could actually sense my organs at work, as though I had opened up a wristwatch to peer at the cogs turning inside. Now and then, a series of what felt like electrical impulses juddered through my uterus, lighting up that dark, wet, under-the-sea cave with what felt like forked flashes of lightening. Such drama. Such mundanity.

The flip-side of all this was illness proper. Disease. The body gone wrong. Its organs working to make something new but disastrous. A cancer rather than a person. This was what Susan Sontag called 'the night-side of life' in her landmark 1978 work *Illness as Metaphor*, written while she was being treated for breast cancer. The essay ruminated on the same theme as Plath in her poem written some two decades earlier, but these two women, both of whom experienced pregnancy and illness, stood on opposite sides of the fence. Plath, the tortured poet, needed metaphor as a sick person needs medicine. Sontag, the firebrand thinker, demanded it be stripped away so we could look at the thing itself. 'The most truthful way of regarding illness – and the healthiest way of being ill – is one most purified of, most resistant to, metaphoric thinking,' she wrote in the essay's remarkable opening paragraphs.

Cancer, she argued, was a 'demonic pregnancy'. A malignant lump, 'a foetus with its own will'. And it was true from the other side too. Pregnancy was a kind of day-side of death. A benign growth that signified a beginning rather than an end. I felt this duality in my newly sensitised body.

Pregnancy and illness were conjoined like birth and death. Two sides of the same coin. Either/or probabilities dicing in my womb. Sontag quoted St Jerome, who, she concluded, must have been thinking of cancer when he wrote, 'The one there with his swollen belly is pregnant with his own death.'

In the months leading up to my discovery of my pregnancy my mother was diagnosed with breast cancer. Another of the body's mysterious acts, though this was one of cruelty rather than kindness. Another growth that could not be controlled. We can grow tumours as weirdly and randomly as babies. My mother's body had achieved both after all. She was a retired doctor who, like most people, had grown more fearful with age, and more patient than doctor. Now the metaphor became reality and the doctor became patient proper. Over the course of a fast and loose year my mother ran the gamut of treatment. An all-too-familiar story with the pace and trajectory of a thriller, delivering plenty of frights, twists and red herrings along the way. It started with a routine mammogram. Something suspicious. Biopsy recommended. The results came quick and were definitive and devastating: cancer.

My mother went on to have a lumpectomy, which uncovered a large, sausage-shaped tumour in her breast. *Sausage-shaped*. These were the very words used by the registrar who came to see us after the operation. My mother lay woozy and elated with post-operative relief in a bed over which hung a sign saying: BED BROKEN. It was funny, that sign. We had to laugh about something. A young woman in the bed opposite who had just had a double mastectomy smacked her lips in thirst as we talked. She was on her own and so I walked over, put a paper cup of water to her mouth, and she drank daintily. Then her eyes filled with tears and she surveyed the room of women in their beds like an actress about to make a thank you speech. Euphoric and drug-addled, she said, 'Such humanity!' and grasped my hand.

Later, my father, sister and I arrived home in a stupefied state to find Claire had made us dinner. Sausage stew, she said. We never laughed at that. We ate it silently in front of the television. There may have been a black humour to this warped picture of familial harmony, but there was something else too. It made me realise, as pregnancy would later do over and over again, that we are capable of making sausage-shaped tumours and babies, and of being turned into sausages too. A nasty, Sweeney Toddish revelation. No wonder we needed to encase it in metaphor to stomach it.

In the end my mother had a mastectomy. She lost a breast, a part of her body that had kept my sister and I alive when we were babies. I remember seeing her after the surgery and looking at the space where her breast had been beneath her hospital gown and thinking a startling thought: I used to suckle there. Why had it never occurred to me before? That my mother gave birth to me, made me in her body, fed me with her body. Such sacrifice and yet so easy to forget. So easy not to know in the first place.

I had no idea how my parents would take my pregnancy. They had two unconventional Indian daughters in their mid-thirties and had probably given up on the likelihood of grandchildren long ago. Arranged marriages were mentioned only as a punchline. Once, the mother of a young doctor back in India – for it was always 'back' whether or not one had ever been there in the first place – had enquired after me, which we all found hilarious. My girls are not the marrying kind, my father would say proudly in one of his Mr Bennet moments. Too independent. Too British.

A dark walk home from work down a long, bleak Edinburgh street with the right angle of Arthur's Seat looming at its southern end and Leith Links to the north. Along the way, a string of old boozers fighting on after the smoking ban with all the stoicism of the men puffing away outside them. I expected their smoke to make my stomach turn but in fact I liked it because it was the smell of my past. It was only a mile from one end of the street to the other and downhill the entire way but walking it was exhausting. I phoned my mother halfway along and spoke those words: 'I've got something to tell you.' The same ones you use when you're telling someone you're ill. That you've got breast cancer.

Instead: 'I'm pregnant.' The word stuck in the throat, as it always did, embarrassing me and stripping me naked for examination. My mother went quiet. 'Oh,' she said. The same 'oh' she'd used, low and noncommittal, when so many years earlier I had run downstairs crying, a balled-up pair of bloodied knickers in my fist. Oh. I knew that 'oh' so well, it turned me back into a child whenever she spoke it. Perhaps it was shock, or her illness, or fear at everything that might yet go wrong, or her own mortality, or something unknown to either of us. Perhaps the plights of mother and daughter, the fact that we were living out the twin possibilities of illness and pregnancy, were too close to bear.

Christmas was a muted affair. My mother reeling from chemotherapy, me from early pregnancy, our malign and benign illnesses proving uneasy festive bedfellows. The result was an interminably long day, heavy with carols on the television and quietness in the room. The sweet, and for me sickly, scent of chicken roasting in cava and apples and the sound of my sister and Claire getting drunk in the kitchen as they cooked. My father in his sagging chair watching the usual stuff: *Ben-Hur*, *Gone with the Wind*. Meanwhile I sat on the sofa watching yet another Christmas, the last one that would ever be like it, go by.

If early pregnancy was in some ways illness in disguise, the symptoms continued to come thick and fast. Constipation one day, diarrhoea the next. Cramps. Sore breasts. The epic tiredness, so soporific and unyielding. The only option was to sink into it. It was almost pleasurable, obeying my body so readily, but there was a sadness too, an understanding that life in all its gloriously policed selfishness would never be the same, that the time for putting up a fight was over. I didn't mind, I welcomed it in fact, but I understood why others felt differently. In the Seventies feminist classic *Fear of Flying*, Erica Jong described pregnancy as an abdication of control, referring to it as a growth inside your body, 'which would eventually usurp your life'.

Next up I developed a vaginal rash that made my skin hot, blistered and itchy. I went to the doctor and was once again instructed to lie on a bed, put my feet together and drop my knees while a speculum was inserted. I had never found this routine remotely painful but for the first time ever my body lashed out in response, felt it as pure invasion. The pain was excruciating, black like a void. I actually screamed out 'No!' and tears sprang to my eyes.

After it was over, I sat watching the GP write out a prescription for steroid cream. The rash was mysterious, like so much in pregnancy, but was possibly a response to heightened hormonal activity. It took months to go away. She asked me about our donor and I felt protective of him, of us, and absurdly afraid of thinking too much about him at all, as if it might somehow transmit to the baby and make it more like him than me. She told me about her three children and recent divorce, information I would never have been party to had I not been pregnant. Pregnancy, I was beginning to understand, made you a vessel not just for your own burgeoning secret but for everyone else's too. People told you things. Life became more intimate inside and out.

She had noticed that lots of women found internal examinations painful during pregnancy. No medical reason for it, she said. In her opinion it was simply because I was carrying 'precious cargo'. Afterwards I walked home through the warren of back streets in Leith, every crooked path eventually leading to the same destination, and thought about the boat bumping across the middle of the Indian Ocean. About carrying precious cargo from one side of the world to the other. I felt afraid of that benign little crescent of sand now. To think of it was to be marooned there once more.

I had experienced this curiously delayed fear once before, after doing a shark dive in, of all places, the Firth of Forth at North Queensferry. Or rather, in an aquarium at Edinburgh's Deep Sea World holding a million gallons of water from the Firth and a handful of sand tiger sharks, cousins of the great white but considerably more slow and placid in temperament. The dive itself, a present from Claire as I had long been obsessed with these magnificent creatures, was exhilarating. Tinkerbell, ten feet of vast, beautifully engineered fish, glided directly above my head in a mirror-image of the reef shark I would swim over in the Maldives. I could have reached out and stroked her smooth white belly if I chose. I was not scared. I felt only the excitement and respect that combine to make awe. It was afterwards that fear came. I would picture myself crouched at the bottom of that tank, small, clumsy and weighted down, as these awesome predators drifted past, silent and remote, mouths partially

33

open to reveal row upon row of teeth, and feel frightened. What was I doing in that unbreathable world? Now I felt the same about the small island approaching the earth's middle. It was a part of the world in which I had no place. 'Often, in my bed at home, I have remembered the places I have run lightly over with no sense of fear and have gone cold to think of them,' wrote the Scottish poet Nan Shepherd about her sensual explorations of the Cairngorms. 'It seems to me then that I could never go back; my fear unmans me, horror is in my mouth. Yet when I go back, the same leap of the spirit carries me up. God or no god, I am fey again.'

I had to be careful with the secret that came everywhere with me now. I couldn't let anyone untrustworthy on board. It was up to me to navigate this journey. There would be illness along the way, as well as loneliness, fear, regret, elation, uncharted waters, the lot. There might be grief. But this was my journey and no one else could make it for me. It was both a comforting and frightening thought, like thinking about the waves pounding the house reef at night. Blackened by the sky. Destined to break and fetch for eternity.

Three

January

Our habitual vision of things is not necessarily right:
it is only one of an infinite number, and to glimpse an
unfamiliar one, even for a moment, unmakes us, but
steadies us again.
   The Living Mountain, Nan Shepherd

At the start of 2007 I travelled to London to interview a
Scottish artist called Alison Watt. She was halfway through
a two-year residency at the National Gallery and was the
youngest artist in its long and hallowed history to win the
coveted position. It had transported her from a modest
studio in an old church hall in Leith, close to where I lived,
to one of the greatest collections of paintings in the world.
An audacious move, and one not entirely unexpected from
an artist who graduated from Glasgow School of Art with a
commission to paint the Queen Mother.

We met in the morning in the National itself, a neoclassical bruiser of a building overlooking a scene so perfectly
composed and representative of itself that it is like a painting, albeit one forever on the move. The smooth expanse
of Trafalgar Square, Landseer's majestic lions, which every
child, woman and man yearns to clamber upon, to stroke
those bronze curls; the pigeons, tourists and of course the
Londoners, an irrepressible people who pride themselves on
always having somewhere to be and knowing the best way

to get there. The National has presided over all this with the cool disinterest of a palace guard for nearly two centuries.

Once inside, I headed away from the grand theatre of the main galleries with their stern guides flanked by brooding European landscapes and countless Annunciations. I was here for something else; the thrill of going backstage, so different from the still and sober enjoyment one gets from standing before a great painting. This was about the actual people who through wars, recessions, arts council feuds and the plodding on of peacetime had devoted themselves to the continuance of a couple of thousand paintings. The mortal protecting the immortal. The fleeting ensuring the permanence of art. It seemed extraordinary that it was mere people who made paintings at all, just as it would strike me, years later, that it was people who made people.

In a way, to live inside a pregnancy was to make one's own work of art. A thing so singular, strange and unknowable in both execution and result. You knew that you had made it, yet in many ways once it was done it had nothing to do with you at all. This could be crushing, I sensed, but also necessary and thus a source of great pride. The artist Louise Bourgeois, who in a remarkably long and varied career made many works about the pregnant body, wrote about this way of viewing ourselves: 'For me, sculpture is the body. My body is my sculpture.' By the Sixties she had started making what became known as her soft sculptures, which struck me as a lovely name for a foetus, suspended in utero like one of Bourgeois's sculptures hanging in a gallery.

In her case, they were beautiful disembodied forms made out of materials such as rubber, latex, cement and plastic. Her preoccupations were always as much with form as substance, with the pregnant body as much as the creature within. Thus her fascination with curves, rotundity, breasts, eggs, hulking great spiders swollen with forbidding sacs, bulging shapes dangling in space, spirals that wound on and on representing both control and freedom, circles and the eternity they promised. And she saw bodies, and her own in particular, as landscapes to be discovered. Bourgeois considered the body 'a land with mounds and valleys and caves and holes', concluding that 'our own body is a figuration that appears in mother earth'.

If our bodies were our sculptures, our very own figurations in mother earth, the pregnant body seemed to me the strangest and most powerful one of all. Here was an act of creation that meant being briefly let into the secret of existence. Invited behind the curtain. Witnessing the marvel of David emerging slowly and spectacularly from an old hunk of marble. It involved inhabiting a different time and space, just as making a work of art does, for already I was talking and thinking in weeks rather than months, a habit that every pregnant woman develops soon enough.

I walked through room after room and down corridor after corridor until I had no idea how I would find my way back out. Fresh paint perfumed the air, the thrilling scent of artists at work. The muffled noises of people, permissible here but still somehow subversive in the altered atmosphere of a gallery. I finally arrived at a studio, small but lofty and bright, which gave it a chapel-like feel, and flooded with the soft yellowing light particular to winter mornings and paintings by Old Masters. In the centre of this lovely composition was Watt, a tiny woman with eyes so blue and piercing they appeared unblinking. She possessed a matching bird-like intensity and was aptly perched upon a paint-spattered scaffold.

Expecting

How to explain the series of paintings she was working on in this remarkable place? They were as vast as she was small, which explained the scaffold, and perhaps as a response to being among so many monumental works of art they were getting bigger. Still, what were they? On one level, they were beautifully rendered close-ups of folds of fabrics, crisp, undulating, crinkled, at once as old as the Renaissance and as achingly modern as an almost blank canvas. On another level, they were just that: nearly nothing at all. Absences. They seemed to me to be holes, or voids, or vaginas. Dark places we are drawn to but cannot understand. They were shape-shifting paintings: abstract and realist, massive and miniaturist, a kind of purist trompe l'oeil. You wanted to enter them, cloak yourself in them, be swallowed up by their cavities just as Alice was by the rabbit hole. I said as much to Watt, that the holes appeared to represent vaginas, and she laughed and replied, 'That says much more about you than it does about me.'

Watt had spent an entire career referencing historical paintings and some of her favourites were pinned to the wall as scrappy cut-out reproductions. One in particular caught my eye. It was Gustave Courbet's *The Origin of the World*. I had never seen this icon of oil painting before. A small, deeply erotic work, it was painted by the French master of realism in 1866, but displays none of the prudery of its time. A time when the pain of childbirth was considered a rite of passage for women and the Old Testament view that 'in sorrow thou shalt bring forth children' still held. Of course, Courbet's masterpiece was shocking then but the true shock of seeing it that morning was that its power of provocation had lingered. There was something about its frankness, its bare-faced cheek, its glorious celebration of women's genitalia as at once pleasure-giving and life-giving. No surprises that the painting was owned for a time by the psychoanalyst Jacques Lacan. It says as much about the origin of our minds as our bodies. It tells us something so obviously true that it becomes shocking: that the origin of the world is the body. The female body as world. Mother nature in her most figurative form.

The painting is a close-up and ruthlessly sensual view of a woman's nude body. We cannot see her face, arms or legs: in magazine parlance, they have simply been cropped out. There is nowhere else to look, no context to soften or distract us from the naked truth of female sexuality and – remember, the work's somewhat ironic title – fertility. She reclines on a bed in a post-coital pose: a single breast with an erect nipple peeping out from a sheet, a hillock of tummy, wide vista of hips, one leg carelessly thrown open to reveal a luscious tumble of pubic hair crowning the full lips of her vulva. The painting is a thing of flesh and warmth and life. It beckons us back into the origin of the world. It invites us to return to the place where we all began.

When paintings affect us, we hold them in our minds and can summon them up at will. Sometimes they don't even need summoning. They simply belong to us, as if our minds were art thieves gadding about stealing great paintings and restoring them into memories. No, they do more than belong to us: they become us and we become them. So we eat out late and alone in a big city and feel we are Edward Hopper's *Nighthawks*. In the bluest well of grief, we cry ourselves into Picasso's *Weeping Woman*.

Something similar occurred when it came to my twelve-week scan. This is the first great landmark in pregnancy, when you discover how 'far along' you are and thus when the baby is due, though this is a notoriously imprecise science. Most remarkable of all, you get to see the baby for the first time. It is the ultimate proof, the first step taken on the moon, with all the thrill, wonder and disbelief one would associate with such a great adventure. Put simply, it is the moment when you allow yourself to think that you are going to have a baby.

For me, a strange kind of displacement happened and a look inside my body became a look at a painting, just as a few weeks earlier it had transmogrified into a look at all the wombs in the world. It started as before, a ritual I had already come to love. The full-to-bursting bladder. The belly of whirling dervishes in the waiting room, this time in a small community treatment centre beside a well-used Victorian baths in Leith. The sense of anticipation, that almost unpleasant brew of emotions that is so easily mistaken for terror.

The sonographer was a rather stern woman who scolded me for forgetting my maternity notes: a blue folder stuffed with mostly empty sections that I hadn't yet learned to cart around with me. She said little and had an expressionless face that I was starting to view as a mark of the profession, like gamblers at poker. She guided her device over the flat ground of my belly, pushing the cold jelly here and there, seeking out sound waves that would result in a picture. And sure enough an image swam on screen. A baby. But first, I saw something else: Courbet's *Origin of the World*. For just a split second I saw a realist painting that, unbeknownst to me, had been in storage in the recesses of my mind for years. There she was, both myself lying back in that room with my top pulled up and my jeans unbuttoned, and Courbet's model, peeping out from beneath the sheet, one leg thrown wide open. And the sheet was painted by Watt: it enveloped the model in its cool white folds. She was the hole at the heart of it. Or rather, we both were.

Then the painting was gone, evaporating like mist burnt away by the sun. I saw with perfect clarity my own soft sculpture.

It lay on its back, fitting as snugly against the wall of my womb as a pea scooped in a pod. A remarkably adult pose for one so new to the business of existence. I could imagine him – for it seemed suddenly and unequivocally a 'him' – clasping his hands behind his head, whistling a happy tune with a blade of grass in his teeth, cloud-watching, blowing smoke rings from another time. It was a stance as recognisable as a smile: indeed it was contentment written in the language of the body.

The head was most noticeable, still comparatively large and taking up a third of its length, which at this stage was still measured from crown to rump. Remarkably, it already had a considerable profile, one I felt I would be able to pick out in a line-up. Big protrusion of forehead, a nose worth noticing, two jutting lips, and the kind of chin one might call determined. His tummy was what I noticed most of all. It was as rotund as a child's drawing of a hill. Louise Bourgeois would have loved its almost absurd circularity.

In 'Scan', a poem from Kate Clanchy's collection *Newborn*, which charts her pregnancy, birth and experience of early motherhood, she writes of the first sight of her foetus. Of seeing on a screen 'some star lit hills, a lucky sky'. I too saw the world in my womb. The foetus's perfect circle of belly reminded me of a favourite hill in Glencoe, one of those examples of nature expressing itself so impeccably as to seem almost unnatural. It is a bulbous land mass, a boil on the face of a pocked moonscape, startlingly smooth, round and elephantine. From a distance it looks friendly, though distance is the great deceiver when it comes to mountains. Approach any hill up close and it becomes unrecognisable, yet this one really does look friendly in a place characterised by such rough and menacing beauty. One sees this hill on the right when travelling north into the Highlands. It is important to approach it from this direction for two reasons: first, the majesty of Glencoe is amplified beyond measure because it gatecrashes the landscape with such swagger after the lunar flatness of Rannoch Moor. Second, the hill comes before the mountains of Glencoe proper and over the years it has become my own unofficial gateway to the Highlands. A foreshadowing of the great drama to come, just as pregnancy could be seen as a rehearsal for life. The prologue of existence.

As we watched in awe, the foetus began to move. One arm raised up, then the other. They began to punch the air in turn. Tiniest of fisticuffs. A boxing match of one. I glimpsed a shadow of umbilical cord, pulsing it seemed, but I couldn't wholly trust what my eyes were seeing. There was nothing to say, or if anything was said I didn't hear it. I was not moved exactly and I'm not sure I understood that this baby was in me. I was merely fascinated like an artist happening upon an old work in the attic and thinking – did I really paint that? It was the curiosity of witnessing so much movement within me yet feeling nothing. I stared at my belly, trying to comprehend those fists working away beneath all those layers of skin, tissue and muscle, trying to travel through them all to peer over the wall of my womb. Impossible. All was as still as Rannoch Moor on a rare clement day.

To think so much had happened in just twelve weeks. Three short months. A quarter of a year. Not that much longer than a school summer holiday, those gloriously elastic periods of time that stretched into oblivion on a haze of blown dandelions and bike rides downhill without brakes. Time slowed down when we were children, sometimes exasperatingly so, but at the very start, before all that, it seemed accelerated like those nature programmes which speeded life up so that a flower blossomed in a heartbeat and clouds scudded across mountain ranges in moments. How swiftly we all began.

Was a life in utero a life in microcosm? One that ended with birth rather than death? A noted seventeenth-century physician and man of ideas called Sir Thomas Browne wrote about this very concept. 'Surely we are all out of the computation of our age, and every man is some months elder than he bethinks him; for we live, move, have a being and are subject to the actions of the elements, and the malice of diseases, in that other world, the truest microcosm, the womb of our mother.' In 1802 the poet Samuel Taylor Coleridge, who became fascinated by the writings of Browne, wrote these excitable words in response: 'Yes! The history of man for the nine months preceding his birth would probably be far more interesting and contain events of greater moment, than all the three score and ten years that follow it.' Overstating it, perhaps, but that morning in a modest room in a local community health centre in Leith, I knew what he meant. I realised the magnitude of the smallest of beginnings: how biology had been keeping busy in the dark and a tiny skeleton had somehow been building itself inside a larger one. And how this went on forever, reaching further back into the past like a neverending procession of Russian dolls. The dizzying view into the bowels of the ocean I had encountered a month earlier. The chicken and the egg conundrum playing out in womb after womb.

Expecting

It was the level of detail in something so small and unfinished. The foetus measured just 6 centimetres, yet already all of its vital organs were in place. I tried to picture a tiny heart, littlest of lungs, and it was like playing with doll's house furniture; beautiful in its meddling with scale but unreal. And yet. The facial bones were formed. Thirty-two tooth buds could be counted. The eyes were fully developed though still widely spaced, like all those noble animals who needed to see the world around them and could do so without having to turn their heads. This would change over the weeks and months to come as the eyes continued on their march forward towards the front of the face. The external ears – known as pinnae, Latin for 'wing' – were unhearing but beginning to take shape. The fingers were now beginning to separate into digits, as were the toes. Nails were already present. The skin remained transparent but now it was covered in the softest, finest layer of down, graduating from octopus to seal. It was permeable too: the amniotic fluid could seep through it like sunlight warming skin.

It was a shock. I was only a third of a way through the journey but to some extent the deed was done. The hardest part was already accomplished, which seemed odd for I had imagined this journey as an ascent, getting harder the further one progressed. But the risks were actually decreasing as I travelled the distance. There was now less than a 1 percent chance of miscarriage. All that was left, for both of us, was to grow and mature. This would happen rapidly, for him, at an alarming rate of half an inch each week. So many great works of art had taken longer to paint, model or write.

We left with a selection of pictures of our own minor masterpiece and a due date for what it was worth: 20 July. 'A perfect baby,' were our taciturn sonographer's parting words.

'The best I've seen this morning.' Perhaps she said this to everyone. No matter. These words were as intoxicating as the praise of any great critic. It was my first rush of pride and it hit hard, just as I hoped those tiny little fists would one day soon. I thought of everything I had accused my body of over the years, how painfully hard I had been on it. It was too skinny, too fat, too voluptuous, too hairy, too dark, too light, too Indian, not Indian enough. My nose was too wide and squashy, my thighs too twig-like, my feet too flat, my stomach not flat enough. My hair was too curly, then it was too straight. I was short-sighted enough to be unable to see the biggest letter on the eye chart and had lived with chronic back and shoulder pain for years. My neck had an excruciating habit of going into spasm, and some mornings the nerves in my arms were so inflamed my little fingers were numb. I had intermittent sciatica in my right leg and a constantly clicking right big toe. My body was a problem – in short, a site to be managed, policed and occasionally ravaged.

In 1980 the American poet Sharon Olds wrote about pregnancy and birth's capacity to enable women to revel in their own bodies. In 'The Language of the Brag,' she confessed: 'I have wanted some epic use for my excellent body / some heroism, some American achievement.' The poem is a gleeful, boastful and incredibly direct riposte to male poets – she names Walt Whitman and Allen Ginsberg specifically – whom Olds felt had seized the act of writing about birth for themselves. Their male voices were so loud and boastful they had drowned out the others. The ones who birthed them. In 'The Language of the Brag', Olds speaks up and reclaims both the act of birth and the act of writing about it for herself and all women. This is how it ends:

Expecting

I and the other women this exceptional
act with the exceptional heroic body,
this giving birth, this glistening verb,
and I am putting my proud American boast
right here with the others.

Seeing that baby relaxing in the hammock of my womb, I realised something for the first time in my life. My body was not a machine that would wear down over time and eventually break. It was a work of art in progress. It had been made by another woman's body and it had brought me to this very moment in time. It was strong enough to have lasted thirty-four years. It could sustain a life for now and, I hoped, for another half a year. Six months. Twenty-four weeks. I was already doing it. For a dizzying moment I revelled in my fertility as a man does his virility. My body started to speak the language of the brag. I swaggered out of there and felt like the origin of the world.

Four
February

... the gestation drive [is] just like the desire to write: a desire to live self from within, a desire for the swollen belly, for language, for blood.

The Laugh of the Medusa, Hélène Cixous

One by one, we went round the room. Each woman introduced herself, divulged how far along she was, and described how she was getting on. One woman's pelvic girdle was in agony, though I had no idea what this meant. I assumed a girdle was a belt as outdated as a corset, had never considered my pelvis before, and was only vaguely aware of its cradle-like shape and its location at the foot of my spine. A memory of skeletons swinging from stands in science class rather than of my own body. A memory that, like a skeleton, now wanted flesh on its bones.

Another woman was still battling sickness five months into her pregnancy. She was a teacher and could barely eat, let alone get up in front of a class five days a week. That morning she had vomited blood into the toilet before work. Others spoke of lower back pain, weird dreams, sugar addictions, swollen extremities, trapped wind, sudden and uncontrollable fits of weeping, an inability to concentrate and, of course, the most classic and unrelenting symptom of all: exhaustion. If you didn't know this was an antenatal yoga class you might be forgiven for thinking you were eavesdropping on an AA meeting.

I noticed something else, too. After each stricken solilo-
quy, the speaker would do a little laugh of self-dismissal. This
would be followed by something along the lines of 'ah well'
or 'never mind' or 'shouldn't complain' or 'apart from that
I'm fine'. So even here, in a space provided solely for them,
these women didn't feel entitled to their own feelings. This
was how dislocated, apologetic and alone we felt. This was
how difficult it was to articulate, let alone bear, the ancient
mysteries of pregnancy and childbirth.

'In woman's womb word is made flesh,' wrote James Joyce
in 'Oxen of the Sun', book fourteen of *Ulysses*. '... but in the
spirit of the maker all flesh that passes becomes the word that
shall not pass away. This is the postcreation.' 'Oxen of the
Sun' is renowned for being the most dense and heavy-go-
ing chapter of Joyce's masterpiece, which seems appropriate
for its subject matter: the long and difficult birth of one
woman's baby and, just as explicitly, of language itself. The
fertility of words and the bodies that invent, speak and write
them. The action takes place in a Dublin maternity hospital,
where Mina Purefoy has already been labouring for three
days, while a group of rowdy, bawdy men ignore her tra-
vails and pontificate about pregnancy, from contraception
to Caesarean sections, in a room down the hall. It's a rol-
licking ride through the gestation of prose in Western liter-
ature, beginning in a staccato Latinate verse and ending in
a sozzled heap of Dublin slang. And this dizzying and often
alienating verbal assault is also an extended metaphor for
what takes place in a pregnancy. Joyce wanted to chart the
gestation of the human embryo through the development of
language. The text is literally pregnant. Nine linguistic styles
(Purefoy's response to her baby, for example, is in Charles
Dickens's sentimental prose) split into nine sub-sections

referencing the nine months spent in the womb. Birth and
death connected by an invisible and everlasting spool of language. In the end, words are all that is left. The sounds in
mouths and marks on pages that outlast each and every one
of us. The postcreation.

As for me, it was as though I had wandered off the street
into a secret meeting to which I hadn't really been invited.
Mine was the earliest pregnancy in the room by a long way
– just sixteen weeks – which made me feel like a little girl in
a room of *grandes dames*. I felt so out of place it may as well
have been a working men's club or a locker room. I was more
like the journalist who had come to write a story on this
group of women than one of them. I felt like an imposter. I
suppose I was in shock, which in pregnancy had a habit of
hitting you twice. First, the thing itself; whatever sensation,
physical or emotional, happened to be tearing through you
at that moment. Then came the aftershock. The having not
known it before. The fact that your own body, the thing that
belonged to you most in the world and perhaps the only
thing you could be said really to possess, had the power to
shock you at all. Time and time again, I heard myself and
other pregnant women voice this. *I can't believe I never knew.*

A neat narrative circle had brought me here, to the Pregnancy and Parents Centre, one of those sleights of hand life
occasionally deals you that shrink the world and turn you
into a character in a Dickens novel. The building itself was
small, ugly and unremarkable, as buildings in which remarkable things happen so often are. Many of the other premises
on the street were working garages, spaces largely associated
with men, where machines rather than bodies were endlessly
worked on, loved and sent back out into the world. An old
canal ran parallel to this road, or rather the end of one, which

was apt considering all the 'birth canals' you would never know were being visualised inside the pregnancy centre. Both were hidden. The one inside me became a canal only when I was pregnant. The other took me weeks to discover, obscured as it was by the inky evenings of February and an old brick wall across the road from the centre. In fact, the Union Canal, which runs from Falkirk and was originally constructed to bring minerals to the capital, had been there since 1822. But no one thought of Edinburgh as a canal city, just as no one thought of it as a city by the sea, or indeed of their vagina as a canal. That is, until pregnancy, as well as planting a foetus in you, imprinted a whole new way of seeing, thinking and talking about your body on your mind. This eastern end of the Union Canal closed in 1921 when the basins were filled in, and now the area, with its smattering of leisure facilities, businesses and building sites forever in progress, had that glassy, unpeopled look of an architectural drawing come to life.

The pregnancy centre was anomalous in this area perpetually on the verge of regeneration. A small and rather shambolic not-for-profit organisation that had been running for more than two decades, it was started up by a gentle but steely woman called Nadine who in the early days ran it from her own living room, providing tea, cake and support for pregnant women planning natural births – the kind of woman-centred environment that was in seriously short supply in the hyper-medicalised Eighties.

I had crossed paths with this woman before. Rewind more than a decade to Glasgow, city of old ships, new shops, highrises, low skies, the best of art, music and attitude and the one that came along when I badly needed a city to call my own. This was where I got my first job as a journalist at *The*

Four • February

Big Issue in Scotland, the magazine sold by and for homeless people. At that time it operated out of a magnificent 1920s building in the Merchant City that was once a telephone exchange. Like so much of Glasgow, its grandeur was somewhat diminished by the wasteland its arched windows overlooked, home to weeds, puddles and the odd car. For those who loved Glasgow – and those who did, loved it ferociously – this chequered beauty was part of its charm.

The first article I pitched to my editor was about home birth. I've no idea why. I was in my early twenties and had no plans to have children, let alone give birth to them at home. I needed to find a pregnant woman to be my first ever interviewee and a sub editor called Tracey, who had also just started at the magazine, suggested I ask a woman who ran a group in Edinburgh and who had been with her during the home birth of her second child. This woman was Nadine. Tracey recalled squatting deeply during the pushing stage of labour, her arms tight around Nadine's body. And Tracey, it turned out, would become my family for she was Claire's sister. The baby was my future nephew.

I remember little of my conversation with Nadine, except that she gave me the number of a pregnant woman who was planning a home birth. I phoned this woman to interview her, my first cold call, heart thudding so loud it seemed to reverberate down the receiver and my little rehearsed speech evaporating from my mind as soon as she answered. She listened patiently to my mumblings and then after a terrible pause told me that she had lost her baby. Only last week. So there would be no interview, she said with devastating matter of factness. She hung up as I was saying sorry. I was shocked at the peek through the curtain of a stranger's private life that journalism had suddenly sanctioned. I felt a certain amount of horror that our lives had collided at all. But I was young, too, and full of the unthinking robustness of youth. Death had not yet touched me, and I don't think I fully understood the tragedy that woman was living, and would live always. By the end of the day I had found another pregnant woman to interview.

Now here I was, more than a decade later, in Nadine's centre, pregnant with a baby Claire and I had conceived in our minds if not our bodies. Now I was the one with the baby inside me, and the one who might lose it too. And now that I was older I understood the cruel blows life could rain down on you. I had felt their force myself. Arriving at the building, I felt the click of coming full circle. These degrees of separation connected us all; they weren't extraordinary, but in pregnancy they seemed to crackle with extra energy. Perhaps this was because the stranger growing inside me was another link in the chain and one that bound me more to the world somehow and all the people born in it. Perhaps this was what the Scottish-American naturalist John Muir was getting at when he wrote: 'When we tug at a single thing in nature, we find it attached to the rest of the world.' Or as Joyce puts it in *Ulysses*, 'The cords of all link back, strandentwining cable of all flesh.' I couldn't stop marvelling at this most fundamental fact of existence, one I realised I had never truly known until now. We had all been born. More than that: 'Life on the planet is born of woman,' wrote the feminist poet and activist Adrienne Rich. We lived our lives so preoccupied with the knowledge of our deaths that our births were forgotten. And once I remembered it, my birth no longer seemed a single event in the past. It became sinewy, alive and continuous, like a river. 'To be alive is to be slowly born,' wrote Antoine de

Saint-Exupéry. 'Human beings are not born once and for all on the day their mothers give birth to them,' wrote Gabriel Garcia Màrquez, 'life obliges them over and over again to give birth to themselves.'

Meanwhile the discussion went on around me. At this stage of pregnancy, one woman asked (I think she was around twenty-four weeks), should she be sleeping on her left side only? A ripple of belly rubs travelled round the room like a murmuration of starlings, a caress that seemed to signify both defence and protection. This was the universal body language of pregnant women, just as you would find skipping children wherever you went in the world. The yoga teacher, Lee, was a fabulously opinionated ex-community midwife with dyed red hair down to her waist. A woman with two grown-up children, both born at home, who told us with some relish that she had eaten her own placenta, thinly sliced in sandwiches, and this in spite of being a vegetarian. She said there was some evidence – and it was only ever 'some' in pregnancy – that sleeping on the left side improved blood flow to the placenta but that it only mattered, if at all, in the final stages of pregnancy. 'Do whatever feels right,' she ordered with a glint of radicalism in her eye that I would come to find deeply reassuring. 'Your body will tell you if it's wrong.'

Nevertheless, when it came to the relaxation session at the end of the class we all obediently flipped onto our left sides with the synchronicity of sunbathers on the beach. Just in case. Pregnant women were easy prey, especially en masse. We were like pods of seals diving in waters patrolled by orcas. The more of us there were, the safer we were. Yet at the same time the danger was greater. The stakes were so high. We all wanted so badly to make it back to shore.

Expecting

Finally, it was my turn. 'Hello, my name's Chitra and I'm sixteen weeks pregnant with my first baby,' I said. 'I'm feeling fine...' I stalled and laughed the same laugh. 'I don't really feel very pregnant compared with all of you.' I couldn't think of anything else to say. Pregnancy was like that: it consumed you night and day, you lived cocooned inside the experience just as the foetus lived inside you, then someone would ask you what it was like and you were stumped. The clichés and inanities took over. You ended up talking about cravings, nursery schemes, birth plans and all the other nice, clean, safe pregnancy topics that papered over the reality. Like a magpie, you started to steal glittering, distracting phrases about pregnancy that others might want to hear and lined your nest with them, using them to protect yourself from a world that seemed increasingly loud, bright, hazardous and out of step with what was happening to you. As with all the deepest, wildest, most difficult experiences, any attempt at explaining pregnancy reduced it, rubbed it out altogether. And so you ended up focusing on the bits that you could comprehend, just as people concentrated on the funeral arrangements instead of the death.

I suspected this was also true of childbirth – more so, for it was an experience engulfed by silence even before it was over. So many mothers I spoke to said they had forgotten their labours, that nature herself had designed it that way to make it more bearable and to enable them to do it again. 'Who can remember pain, once it's over?' wrote Margaret Atwood in her chilling dystopian novel *The Handmaid's Tale*. 'All that remains of it is a shadow...' It was true. No one seemed able to articulate what a contraction really felt like. In fact, they said it was impossible to describe the feeling. I had never heard a full account of labour. The language, like

Joyce's chopped-up slang at the end of 'Oxen of the Sun', always seemed to falter and break down.

In the Seventies the French theorist and feminist Hélène Cixous gave this unacknowledged gap between women's experience and language's inability to describe it a name: *'écriture féminine'*. 'Woman must write her self,' she urged in her landmark essay *The Laugh of the Medusa*, 'must write about women and bring women to writing, from which they have been driven away as violently as from their bodies.' She wrote about the gestation drive resembling the desire to write. So my pregnant body *was* my text, and now I needed to summon the words to write it. It was Joyce's 'postcreation' (and indeed Cixous called *Ulysses* a perfect example of *écriture féminine*) all over again.

Just as the language needed to be rewritten, the response to childbirth was inadequate too. It was more often prurience than genuine interest. People thirsted for blood and drama and resolution. Childbirth was pregnancy's greatest mystery and fear and, like death, perhaps this was because no one really wanted to hear the truth of it. It brought them too close to the precipice of existence.

It made me think of a Vietnam veteran I once interviewed. A wholesome, immaculately dressed and highly decorated man called Karl who had the squarest of shoulders and a side parting so sharp it looked as though it had been achieved with a ruler. We met in the lobby of a swanky hotel in Bloomsbury, as incongruent a setting as you could muster for a discussion about war and death. I have never seen anyone tremble the way Karl did. The man was a living earthquake. His body convulsed inside his beautiful pinstripe suit, his hands shook even when he pressed his fingers together in an attempt to quieten them, his lips wobbled, the muscles in his face twitched.

Still, he talked. He told me that when he returned from Vietnam he spoke to no one about what had happened. He said this dispassionately, as though it could not have been any other way. 'There is a silence that's required,' he explained. 'If you talk about the bad things you're whining and if you talk about the good things you're bragging. Society has very conveniently worked out how to shut everyone up about this.' Childbirth bore no relation to war trauma yet there was something about the response – this deadening of truth – that was comparable. Society did have a way of silencing people, and particularly women, who had seen, felt or lived something vast and irreducible. This was part of what Rich called 'the theft of childbirth from women'. The very words had been stolen from our mouths, the experience snatched from our bodies.

War, birth and death had something else in common. They were all stripped back and unadorned experiences that revealed something about ourselves – often unpalatable – that was raw, unfiltered and existed in this bottomless place beyond language. This was how the African American writer Toni Morrison, whose novels are written in the most sensuous *écriture féminine*, put it: 'Birth, life, and death – each took place on the hidden side of a leaf.'

At the end of the yoga class, the leaf momentarily blew over and I saw its delicately veined underside. My first encounter with the truth of childbirth. It would happen now and then at the end of the yoga class; a woman would attend with her newborn and tell her labour story while the rest of us sat around her in a circle, the most receptive of audiences. I would come to get used to these thundering dramatic monologues, each one worthy of a spotlight and a stage. But this was the first, and it shook me to my core.

The story was not itself seismic in the canon of labour stories, which tended to be as gripping, labyrinthine and slippery as any Shakespearean tragedy. They were often relayed
by narrators as unreliable as a protagonist in a modernist
novel. This was because memory, like time and language,
played tricks on you in moments of great drama. And there
was no drama greater than birth.

The woman, whose newborn girl mewled in her arms as
she spoke, had a natural birth in a pool at the Lothian Birth
Centre, a midwife-led unit adjoined to the Royal Infirmary
that had opened a few years previously. She spoke of the long
wait at home until she and her partner deemed it the right
moment to go to hospital. I learned that this was when the
contractions were a few minutes apart and lasting roughly a
minute but I still couldn't remotely understand what these
casually spoken words signified. It was like trying to comprehend the length of a light year. My mind could no more
conjure up a series of contractions than it could conceive of
the distance between two stars in a galaxy.

She went on to discuss the arc of labour, how what was
known as the 'first stage' was the most difficult because it
seemed it would never end. Someone asked how long this
period lasted and she said she could not remember but it
was hours. She had wanted to get into the birthing pool
early on to relieve the pain but her midwife wouldn't let
her as she wasn't dilated enough. Eventually she had defied
her, jumped in anyway (this pleased Lee greatly), and things
started to progress. The second stage, the only one that
ever made it into cinematic accounts of childbirth, was not
as bad as she had expected. The baby was born with a few
gigantic pushes. Afterwards, before she birthed her placenta,
she wandered around the room dragging her umbilical cord

behind her like a leash. We all laughed at this description but the image of it stayed with me for a long time. I was afraid of it. It seemed too animalistic, too far removed from the soft focus and deliberately unspecific image of childbirth I had subconsciously constructed over the years.

Still, childbirth remained far away enough to seem unimaginable, and sometimes at night, with my hand resting on my rising and falling belly and my eyes wide open, unimaginably frightening. Inside me the work continued, instructed by nature's invisible hand. The baby was now the size of an avocado and growing at the rate of Alice in Wonderland on one of her potions. Over the next few weeks alone it would double in weight. Its sex was becoming clearer. Its facial bones were complete. For the first time its hands could meet across its body as its arms had lengthened; it could reach out and grasp the umbilical cord. The eyes had now moved to the front of the head, the ears were approaching their final position and could hear for the first time. The heart, small and industrious, was pumping twenty-five quarts of blood every day. The foetus could make facial expressions – a rudimentary frown or grimace – and move its eyes behind scrunched lids. It could sense changes in light outside the womb. It could hear music. And it had fingerprints, which in the eyes of society gave it an identity of its own.

A major change had taken place in the role of the amniotic fluid. I imagined this as the softest and most silken of waters, like a calm sea at dusk when the sun has warmed it almost to the same temperature as your body and it feels so limpid against your skin it's hard to tell where the water ends and you begin. When you swim in such waters they thicken like milk and hold you in the softest of embraces. In the first trimester the amniotic fluid had been absorbed through the foetus's skin, like light, but now the kidneys were starting to work and the baby was swallowing the fluid, like water. It would then be excreted back into the sac, absorbed and replaced over and over again, a bath forever being drained and rerun.

But to be honest I still wasn't thinking much of the baby. Not yet. I hadn't felt it move inside me. My stomach still belonged to me. It was too early to buy things, consider names. Even picturing it was a peculiarly disengaging activity. I would look at the small series of scan photos we had and the more I looked, the less they belonged to me. They started to look the same as all the images I had seen over the years, proudly pinned to fridge doors or kept in the wallets of friends. It was like saying a word over and over again until it lost all meaning. Or finding the source of a river and realising that instead of understanding it more, it only became more mysterious. There was no unlocking this kind of mystery. You could merely revel in it. The Scottish modernist poet and writer Nan Shepherd, whose stone slab lying in a small court outside Edinburgh's Writer's Museum simply states 'It's a grand thing to get leave to live', wrote about this idea in *The Living Mountain*, her only non-fiction book. 'I have seen its birth,' she wrote of watching the power and movement of water in the Cairngorms, 'and the more I gaze at that sure and remitting surge of water at the very top of the mountain, the more I am baffled.' This was how I felt about the birth of the foetus inside me, and increasingly about my own birth too.

The Living Mountain, completed in 1944 but not published for more than thirty years, was a book I kept returning to during my pregnancy. Even the title became a kind of metaphor for pregnancy, though the mountain referred not to the body but to the Cairngorm massif, which Shepherd spent a lifetime loving and walking, often barefoot on a sprung floor of heather. It was Shepherd's way of seeing, of wanting to circle a mountain, touch it, live alongside it, rather than climb or conquer it, that spoke to me. It seemed the ideal way to approach the journey of pregnancy. Hers was an *écriture féminine* of the land: Shepherd chose to walk it, and indeed write about it, in the same cyclical, non-linear way that Cixous urged women to write in the 'white ink' of their milk ... 'not about destiny, but about the adventure of such and such a drive, about trips, crossings, trudges, abrupt and gradual awakenings, discoveries of a zone at once timorous and soon to be forthright'.

I wanted to do the same. To resist the sense of countdown, of wishing each moment away, of marking off the days and weeks in the way that so characterised pregnancy. The fact was that the end of gestation was so powerful it obliterated the means. Pregnancy became the opening act and birth the main draw. This was why, whenever I told a mother about one of my pregnancy symptoms, her response inevitably began 'just wait until...' It annoyed me. I didn't want to wait. I didn't want to look ahead. Like Shepherd, I wanted to stop. Look down. To feel my feet pressed to the hill. To squat and plunge my hands into it whenever I wanted.

I was beginning to feel the bloom associated with this golden trimester of pregnancy. The one after the sickness and before the enormity. The one in which the wombfruit (as Joyce called it, knocking the words of the Bible over so they stood on their head) began to ripen. The most notable evidence of this was my breasts, which seemed to swell overnight with the promise of milk. A map of blue veins sketched itself over them and my areolas, the halo circling each nipple, expanded and darkened like pupils dilating in the night. Looking at them in the mirror was a dissociating experience for they looked like the breasts of a mother. The woman I had yet to become. My body was disseminating the biological information faster than my mind.

The strangest symptom of all seemed at first to have nothing to do with pregnancy. Each day I would wake up and find it increasingly painful to open my mouth. It was as though an imaginary hand was clamping my jaw shut through the night so that in the morning my mouth felt old and dusty, like a drawer that hadn't been opened in years. It was as if it needed oiling. It ached as though it longed to speak the secrets of pregnancy; my body seemed to be responding in the most literal of ways to my inability to open up and talk. Eventually I went to see my dentist, who had just had her first baby. She told me the same thing had happened to her and that she had treated many pregnant women with stiff jaws. 'You bite down too hard in the night,' she explained. 'Pregnant women do this. You're tired and nauseous and probably worried about what's coming.' I found this hard to believe. I didn't even feel that stressed. And yet. I thought of my breasts, how they were already streets ahead of my mind. Perhaps my jaw was working something out too, chewing on secrets in the night. Things now seemed to be happening inside me without my knowledge or say-so: a split was taking place between mind and body that was so visceral I could feel rather than understand it. The dentist measured my mouth for an NHS guard to wear at night but by the time it was ready for collection a fortnight later my jaw had mysteriously eased.

At the end of my sixteenth week, I had a midwife appointment. My midwife, Sarah, was young, newly qualified and from the tiny, monastic island of Iona. I adored her. She was refreshingly untainted by the ongoing battles of midwifery and not yet jaded by the splutter and creak of the NHS. She loved attending home births and spoke about how wonderful it was to just sit back and watch the woman get on with it. And I liked the fact that she did not yet have her own children. She seemed in awe of childbirth in the way that only someone who had yet to do it but saw it up close and regularly could be. The appointment began, like the others that would follow, with a ritual as rigorous and comforting as a child's bedtime routine. A blood pressure check, urine sample, blood tests if necessary, a measurement of my bump and a 'listen in' to the baby's heartbeat.

We spoke about my due date, 20 July, which I felt was too early. After all, I knew precisely the moment when I had conceived. Also my menstrual cycle was long, which meant I was likely to have a longer gestation. I wanted to change my due date to 22 July, which seemed like splitting hairs, but I sensed that time would slow down towards the end and I might be grateful for those two extra days. Sarah changed the date without any further discussion. I was lucky. I spoke to a number of women who had also tried to change their due dates under the perfectly reasonable proviso that they knew their bodies better than anyone else. They had been denied this simple agency, a few of them on the Orwellian grounds that 'the system' had calculated the date accurately from their twelve-week scan and it could not be changed.

Finally I lay on the narrow bed and Sarah moved a Doppler over my belly, the same device that would be used to monitor the baby during labour. Whenever she did this at these appointments, she would look skywards as I looked at her, an intriguing sequence of expressions flickering across her face as though she were a great actor enjoying a close-up. Absorption, expectancy and just the slightest glimmer of a smile. I wondered whether she would always make this face or whether it was just because it was still new. Either way, I loved the reassurance it gave me. There was something so maternal about it, which was strange considering Sarah was much younger than me.

And then she found what she was seeking. The relief was huge – I don't think I had realised how worried I was that she would find only a vacuum of silence. Instead, so much mischievous noise. We listened to the baby's heartbeat, smiling giddily at one another. It sounded very rapid and light, like the heartbeat of a field mouse. But it was strong, too, and almost alarmingly certain of itself. As the Doppler pressed firmly into my uterus, the heartbeat quickened or slowed like a dance partner following the lead. Sarah explained this was the baby moving, getting excited, responding to her poking and prodding. It kept trying to dance away from her.

The foetus's heartbeat was 140 beats per minute, twice as fast as my own. Over the months to come it would slow as the foetus grew, just as in life we slow with age. So this was the life in microcosm that had moved Coleridge, the nine months that were a rehearsal for the work-in-progress of life. Hearing the baby's heartbeat for the first time, the leaf turned over again and I was briefly permitted another look. To dwell on the mystery of living with two heartbeats knocking out their rhythms inside me. Could they hear one another? Did they communicate inside my body like siblings whispering in bed after lights out? What secrets did they speak? And would my heart get lonely when it was all over? I did not know how to articulate any of this, could barely understand how to feel it. I could only listen in. Afterwards, as I slid off the table and returned to my seat to agree a date for our next appointment, I felt the almost imperceptible change in the wind as the leaf flipped back over again.

Five

March

Leaning back on the railway wall,
I tried to remember;
but even my footprints were being erased
and the rising stars of Orion
denied what I knew: that as we were
hurled on a trolley through swing doors to theatre
they'd been there, aligned on the ceiling,
*   ablaze with concern*
for that difficult giving,
before we were two, from my one.
Thaw, Kathleen Jamie

A couple of years before I became pregnant, I experienced my first death. Claire's father, a man as small and spry as a mouse, fell ill one autumn. Andy never appeared unwell aside from the habit he had of blowing his nose, which he did excessively with a handkerchief produced from his pocket, and more out of nerves than necessity. His body's engine ran on tension. A small spot of eczema covered the furrow of his brow and flushed red whenever he was especially worried. He was a man who loved to walk quickly and methodically whether in city or countryside, always looking like a person with a destination in mind. This too was about outpacing his anxiety, only this time walking it off was not an option.

We learned in the roundabout way common to families that he had lost his appetite. This in itself was not so unusual.

Andy lived alone, surrounded by model ships and a table perpetually set for tea at which one never saw him eat. He had a passion for cookery books that living alone had permitted to escalate into a fully grown obsession and that had little to do with the actual business of cooking. Or, indeed, eating. These books filled every shelf, which in turn covered every wall, and like a character in a novel Andy sat in the midst of his fragile house of leaves, consuming words in place of the delights they promised. Actually, he didn't cook much at all. He was the kind of man you would spot around Edinburgh rather than at his stove at teatime, propped up at the window of one of his favourite pubs, drinking a pint of lager. On his own, always. A quick hello, generally enacted silently through the glass, and then we would move on. He didn't want company, it was said. He was a man who liked drinking, walking, living on his own. It turned out the only activity he didn't want to do by himself was dying.

When the diagnosis of late-stage oesophageal cancer came, it was impossible to tell how long Andy had been experiencing symptoms. One imagined he had not been eating for weeks because the tumour in his oesophagus was so big the doctor could not get the endoscope past it to examine his stomach. Perhaps his throat hurt, his stomach was upset, he felt nauseous, or tight-chested. Perhaps he began to wake up panic-stricken in the morning and went to bed ravenous and drunk at night, a jumble of recipes and beer swilling in his concave stomach. We never would find out. These were not the questions to pose, not then, and certainly not later. There was no time for the past, despite the prospect of no future crying out for its memories more than ever. Instead, what needed to be asked, as relentlessly as a child on a long journey, was what next? Where do we go from here? Are we there yet?

Expecting

Within a few weeks we were there and wanted only to go back. The cancer was aggressive and too far gone. The dreaded word 'inoperable' was used. Shrinking the tumour with chemotherapy would only weaken him faster. It was too late for everything. Andy was given a few months to live, if that's what you call it. He died the following March.

Now here I was, a few years on, beginning to visibly brim with the beginning of life. March had come round again and I was finally, proudly, sometimes shyly beginning to show. The period of cradled secrecy was over, and now that time of soporific sickness and its accompanying sense of walking on eggshells within one's own body formed a thick coating of nostalgia. This was a trick of pregnancy: I found myself able to enjoy its quirks and charms most in hindsight.

I was carrying the foetus openly now and had entered what was often termed the 'golden trimester of pregnancy'. A time of blooming, growing, ripening, glowing, and what I presumed was an abundance of cliché as much as of hormones. That becalmed and luminous face of pregnancy, the one you encountered on magazine covers and in leaflets strewn around doctors' surgeries that was as lifeless an image of vitality as one could summon up. The woman soft-faced and serene with one hand resting upon the fecund swell of her stomach. Her womb belonging to the world. Desireless, hairless, hermetically sealed, almost like a baby herself. All that was round, smooth, benign and remote. I could not relate to her. We had nothing in common apart from the obvious. Where was the fear, sadness, hardness, madness, illness, stress, itching, chafing, heat, pain, rage, flatulence, bewilderment and roaring, insatiable need?

On the other hand, now that I was experiencing this from the inside I discovered the beatific state wasn't entirely fiction. I really was feeling soft, radiant and foolishly in love with the world. The same foetus that had stolen my strength was giving it back to me, breathing its own life into my body. A kind of internal resuscitation was taking place.

My hair stopped falling out. I would wash it in the shower and gaze at the plughole with the forensic fascination we reserve for observing our own bodies, watching as the water drained away without a single strand sucked under with it. My eyes and teeth shone an opalescent white, thick, strong and luxuriant as marble. My body felt rich with iron as though I was gorging daily on bloody steak, and my skin felt downy as if I was indeed not just growing a newborn but growing into one myself. My breath became more shallow as my uterus jostled with my lungs for space, making me feel as fragile as a corseted Victorian lady. Weirder still? I liked it. Where before I had enjoyed my body's strength, now I was charmed by its weakness. I wanted it to yield further still, to soften like ripe fruit. I wanted to be preserved like a butterfly wrapped in cotton and kept in a box by a child, taken out now and then to be stroked by tiny, curious fingers.

My belly seemed to push out further by the day, smooth and taut as an egg. My skin stretched with uncomplaining ease, though my lower back groaned at the extra weight and I found myself drooping over anything in my path to relieve it, from dry stone walls to clothes horses. The linea negra, meaning 'black line' in Latin, started to show faintly, as if beneath tracing paper, decorated with the occasional baby hair. It bisected my stomach like a ring around a planet or a veined streak of quartz encircling a pebble. Evidence of a disturbance within. Some mysterious ancient change. Meanwhile, winter was finally departing and clumps of cro-cuses began to push their way out of the hard earth on

Expecting

Leith Links, looking like newborns with their slumped, bedraggled heads.

Walking down the street, I felt an unspoken kinship that I recalled because I had experienced it once before. It was the sensation I'd had when Andy was dying, of acquiring a temporary passport to the land of the terminally ill. Of suddenly being able to tune into death's high-pitched squall, just as you see a postbox only when you need to send a letter. The noise was deafening but only others in the know seemed to hear it. I recalled a friend who had ovarian cancer talking about her newly acquired ability to determine which of the strangers around her in wigs, hats and headscarves were undergoing chemotherapy. All of the grief, pain and precarious tragedy, the shocking ease with which people disappear off the face of the earth and those around them continue, the dark knowledge that's usually hemmed in by the simple going about of one's blissfully uneventful life, was suddenly on display.

And people were beginning to look at me, comment ('that's definitely a boy you've got in there!', 'how far along are you?'), and sometimes even reach out and touch. It could be invasive, moving, unsettling. It could also feel like a responsibility, as though by the mere act of growing a foetus I was being stewarded by the world, even policed, and thus had no choice but to stop and hear its secrets. One day a woman grabbed me by the wrist at the foot of Leith Walk and told me about her miscarriages with her thumb pressed hungrily to my pulse. On another occasion a colleague with whom I rarely spoke emailed me, after spotting my rounded silhouette across the building, to tell me she had lost a baby at four months and now, at forty, had come to terms with the fact that she was never going to have children.

How people stared, particularly women, with a deep, almost male gaze that bore an unnerving resemblance to lust. I began to realise that they weren't really looking at me at all. To be pregnant was to be a kind of mirror. Women, especially, wanted to see themselves in you. At your most visible you became invisible, reflective, your identity shrinking as you grew. I was a living biography, but the story my body appeared to be writing wasn't only mine. My womb was expanding to accommodate the world as much as the foetus. The French philosopher Voltaire wrote that 'the present is pregnant with the future' and I began to feel I was pregnant with everyone else's too. And their pasts. I could sense all the tales of mothers, babies, pregnancies, labours, miscarriages, abortions, infertilities, stillbirths and deaths unfurling around me. It was an exhausting, intense and revelatory way to live. And now the passport was returned to me and though this time the destination was birth, still I felt uneasy. How could it be so close to death? Why had I assumed in the first place they were separated by the continent of a life?

Part of my death preoccupation was created by my twenty-week scan. Also known as the anomaly scan, this is when the sonographer checks the baby for all sorts of defects, running through its organs with the hyper-efficiency of a supermarket assistant checking out groceries, taking measurements of the baby's head, abdomen and thigh bone. It's also when you can find out the baby's sex, though the answer is by no means definitive and it may not be identifiable on the day. No matter. I remained convinced I was having a boy.

I had felt so confident about my twelve-week scan, but now I looked back on my bravado as I looked back on my teenage self: with amusement, embarrassment and a certain amount of wistfulness. I was further into the business of pregnancy now and just as our fears multiply as we age, I had more reasons to fret. And so we returned to the Leith Community Treatment Centre, bigger, older and increasingly nervous, clutching our blue folder again. Our sonographer was a Geordie woman with a softer, more soothing voice than the previous one. I lay back, lifted my clothes and marvelled at the proud hump of my stomach as though I was seeing it for the first time. The cold jelly was applied, and I balked again at the mildly offensive pressure of something hard-edged and manmade pushing into the dome of my flesh.

The following twenty minutes passed in a blur of tiny, mind-blowing, explosive details: a series of fireworks set off in a business-like manner that only heightened their impact. Everything seemed to happen so quickly. There was no time to marvel at the perfect skeleton that had built itself in a dark chamber of my body. There was no time even to listen. The sonographer would touch down on an organ and say 'and there's the...'; sparks would begin to fly, and I would disappear into a trance. By the time I came out of it, she was on to the next one. I found myself unable to keep up with the workings of my own body, pretending to hear what she was saying, politely simulating relief, awe, even interest as the foetus's heart, kidneys, spine, head, fingers, toes and so on were pronounced healthy, in the right place, size and number.

It was like trying to spot fish from the surface of a murky pond. Every now and then a flicker of movement at the periphery of your vision, a release of bubbles, the possibility that your eyes are deceiving you. A network of fine bleached bones that made up the baby's spine and ribs and looked like the most delicate of antique birdcages. The umbilical cord hung untidily like a cable. A head filled with two butterflied halves of a brain. A pulsing heart, strong as a fist. It was like glimpsing fragments of a dream in that there was no trajectory and none of it made sense. There was a lurking feeling that I might be inventing everything I was seeing. Yet all of it felt unquestionably true. The images were less clear than I expected, and much less clear than those of my twelve-week scan, but that seemed fitting. The foetus was becoming less known to me, less made of me, over time. It was as completely divorced from anything to do with me as the skeleton of a dinosaur.

At some point during this bizarre excursion into my uterus, the sonographer's expression changed. 'Is everything OK?' I asked, surprised at how quickly I responded to this shift. My heart was suddenly pounding with the proximity of catastrophe. This was how swiftly, easily and definitively it could all go wrong. 'You have a low-lying placenta' she said. *Low-lying*. The word carried me to the Orkneys, those low-lying islands hunkering down in the North Sea that the poet George Mackay Brown described as 'sleeping whales ... beside an ocean of time'. A very pregnant image. I had no idea that a placenta could lie low like land. Once again, my body had stumped me. The sonographer explained: my placenta was lying low across my cervix, covering it as a plug stops a hole. If this continued to be the case – a condition known as placenta praevia – I would need to have a C-section as there would be a pronounced risk of bleeding and shock if I tried to give birth naturally. My hopes were dashed. I wanted desperately to have a natural birth. The thought of knowing, at this early stage, that the baby would be plucked from my belly as a plant is pulled from the earth, that I would feel nothing at all, was shocking. While I still could not picture myself in the act of giving birth, neither could I imagine myself in a theatre, numb from the waist down.

The sonographer assured me that the vast majority of low-lying placentas rose as the uterus ballooned, changing position without themselves moving. I pictured it tracking the waxing of my womb as a spacecraft orbits the moon. I pictured it stubborn as a limpet, immovable from its life-long position on an ocean-smashed rock. The odds were in my favour and I was booked in for another scan at thirty-two weeks – a lifetime away, as far as I was concerned – to check its mysterious progress.

There was one question left to ask and both Claire and I had agreed long before that we wanted to know the answer. Could she see the baby's gender? 'Yes,' she said, but it seemed the most noncommittal of affirmatives. It was the most ambiguous yes I had ever encountered. I almost felt she was humouring us. Claire and I held hands and I started to sweat profusely. My pulse roared as though it was a river pounding its aggressive course through my system, filling each organ up as it went, bursting the banks of my veins, turning the creases of my palms into rivulets. Pure adrenaline working on a resting pregnant body; the strangest of sensations. I heard myself telling the sonographer in a light, conspiratorial tone, which gave nothing of this turmoil away, that I had long been convinced I was having a boy. 'Hmmmm,' she said, looking at the monitor with the most curious of half-smiles. 'I think you're probably right.' And that was that. We probed no further. She offered nothing more. And throughout the rest of my pregnancy, as I began to imagine this boy more clearly and definitively with each passing day, those five words continued to haunt and amuse me. They seemed so confoundedly unclear. I took them to heart with such certainty.

None of this reassurance stopped me from thinking about death. Expecting life seemed to warrant it. I had reached the midpoint of my pregnancy. I was still a few weeks away from the legal abortion limit in the UK. I felt invested in what was happening to me as one is by the time one is halfway through a walk. I felt that same sense of 'no turning back', that sinking feeling of realising the depth of one's own feelings, the commitment to see it through to the end. I'd boarded Plath's train and there was no getting off. And something else: I was developing a creeping distrust of what had already been, as though my footprints were being rubbed out as I walked. I was carrying the peculiar weight of uncertainty one has on a walk, which WG Sebald notices in *The Rings of Saturn*, his novel excavating the recesses of Suffolk and his own beautiful mind. At the end of a day spent tracing the coastline between Lowestoft and Southwold, Sebald looks back at the 'deserted stretch' he has just covered and notes, 'I could no longer have said whether I had really seen the pale sea monster at the foot of the Covehithe cliffs or whether I had imagined it'.

I had experienced this doubt on a walk many times. It had happened to me most memorably on the long walk to Sandwood Bay on Scotland's brutally exposed north-western tip. The sort of walk that is laid out before your eyes as clearly as any Ordnance Survey map so you can see exactly where you are going and where you have been. Miles of the bleakest moorland, which, on the day Claire and I walked it, was flattened by a gale straight off the North Atlantic so fierce that the rain it carried in its lungs struck our faces like shards of glass. Two lochs had burst their banks, burying the stepping stones through them in inches of icy water so that we had to remove our boots, wade through the drowned landscape, then lie on our backs and wave numbed feet in the wind to dry them off. The further we walked, the worse the weather became and with each boggy step, turning back seemed less and less of an option. The track grew less rather than more travelled as we walked it. We could see it snaking far ahead, and somewhere out there was the lighthouse at Cape Wrath, the most north-westerly point of Britain. Looking back was no more convincing. It was as unknown as what lay ahead, as though our footsteps had been sucked back into the moor. No, we did not stop right there for our first glimpse of the bay backed by giant sand dunes, a freshwater lagoon and the ruins of a house said to be haunted by the ghost of a ship-wrecked seaman. No, we did not lie there and wave frozen feet in the air. What had only just happened became inconceivable. Perhaps this explained our constant need to photograph our experiences: not just to preserve them but to prove to ourselves that we had them in the first place. Now I felt the same about my pregnancy. I doubted my own presence in it. I couldn't project myself into what lay ahead or what had been. And perhaps this explains why Claire started to take photographs of my expanding body every month.

In 1932 the Mexican painter Frida Kahlo made a magnificently macabre work that dwells on birth and death. Kahlo began *My Birth* as two actual events occurred in her life that morbidly entwined both beginning and end. She started the painting after a miscarriage and finished it not long after the death of her mother. So *My Birth* turns out to be about two deaths. Much of Kahlo's work, and indeed her life, was a *danse macabre* between these twin possibilities. She was a woman, after all, who kept a pickled foetus in a jar by her bedside, gifted to her by her doctor. A commemoration of life that was also a *memento mori*. And the origin of her creative life was a death of sorts. The tram crash that nearly killed Kahlo at the age of eighteen was a terrible foretaste of the reproductive traumas that would plague her life: the iron railing that entered her left hip exited through her vagina in a horrific antithesis of birth. Her pelvis was fractured and she was never able to live without pain, walk without a stick or carry a baby to term. Three attempted pregnancies ended in miscarriage, termination and grief. Yet it was this same accident that gave birth to Frida Kahlo the artist. No birth without death; no death without birth.

In *My Birth*, Kahlo depicts the moment of her own birth in the style of a Mexican 'ex-voto retablo', traditionally a token of gratitude to the saints. Yet the scroll at the bottom of the work remains empty. The inarticulacy of childbirth prevails and only the image can speak. So what does it say? Kahlo's oversized newborn head, identifiable by those trademark luscious eyebrows, spills out of her mother's vagina onto a bed stained with blood. Her mother's head is covered with a sheet, as in death. She is an overwhelmingly passive figure, lying prostrate with her legs wide open as the birth happens to her. This is no active scene of childbirth. It is more like the bloody aftermath. Overlooking the curiously static scene is a small painting of the Virgin of Sorrows, weeping in silent dignity as Kahlo so often depicted herself in portraits. In her diary she wrote that in this painting she not only imagined her own birth, she gave birth to herself. Today the painting is owned by the pop star Madonna, an artist whose own career was born out of her mother's death when she was six years old.

Expecting

I understood *My Birth*'s death wish now. To invite the deep breath of life into your body was to beckon its flip side. To wait for a sign of life, as I was now doing as faithfully and anxiously as a mother checking on her breathing newborn, was also to fear a life stilled. For it was around this time that we expect the baby's first movements to be felt. The questions came first. Have you felt the baby move? What does it feel like? Does it hurt? Is it weird? It seemed to be regarded as an apex of pregnancy and was one of the experiences I hungered for the most. Perhaps this was because of the fundamental otherness of it, but it also seemed to be a manifestation of anxiety. While I helplessly waited to feel the baby move, I experienced the nervous charge of it not moving. I kept remembering my scans: all that shifting about, 'those first foetal footfalls, the kneading of sole against womb-wall, turning ... like astronauts in black space' as the nature writer Robert Macfarlane puts it. And yet, all that stillness on the outside. All that lack of evidence of life on another planet.

The first movement is known by the romantic name of quickening, from 'quick', originally meaning alive. These first stirrings have for centuries been used, legally and socially, to determine a foetus's right to life. And the quickening standard must be the most emotional one. Life's first rude kick in the stomach. The moment when the foetus is felt not just inside your body, but moving independently of it. I loved the slipperiness of the word. Hearts could quicken with life and lust, but they could also quicken towards death. A nail bitten to the quick was reduced to its essence, to its absolute nail-ness. And quickening seemed to have its own incantatory power, as though merely speaking the word could bring something back to life. 'The mistress which I serve quickens what's dead,' says Ferdinand in Shakespeare's *The Tempest*.

Quickening seemed to illustrate the uneasy truth that both birth and death were manifestations of life. Their bookending of life did nothing to diminish their closeness, their cruel reflection of one another. Birth pangs and death throes. From childbed to deathbed. Womb to tomb. Labour ward to hospice. Both places full of life and death in equal measure, because to bear witness to either state was to teeter on the precipice of the two experiences. The pregnancies that fizzled out into the smallest and most silenced of deaths. The fact that whatever was born would die. The dying reduced to babes with mouths hanging open. Newborns suspicious and creased as old men.

It seemed no coincidence that the year Kahlo painted *My Birth* was the one in which she produced one of her most famous works, *Henry Ford Hospital*, a disturbing vision of the miscarriage she suffered in a Detroit hospital. In it she surrounds herself with six objects mourning a birth that became a death, and a death that became a painting. Each one is attached to her by a livid red umbilical cord: an orchid, snail, cast of a female torso, fractured pelvis, medical contraption and the foetus that would never be. Meanwhile Kahlo is splayed in the middle of a gigantic bed, adrift on a sea of pain, the floating Frida of so much of her work, detached from the faraway reality of hospitals and a world where miscarriages are a fact of life and everyone dies. Connected only to the death inside her living body.

As I waited for the baby to move, for my own body to do something it didn't know how to do, I kept reliving Andy's final weeks as he was moved into a hospice in Edinburgh, high on a hill overlooking the Firth of Forth. St Columba's opened in 1977 as Scotland's first modern unit dedicated to the care of the dying. Apart from a brief spell away, it has been based in the original Georgian building, which was once called Challenger Lodge, ever since. Challenger Lodge was given its title by Sir John Murray, the father of modern oceanography, who named it after his four-year voyage aboard *HMS Challenger* in the 1870s, the aim being to discover new lifeforms in the deep seas. The Challenger Expedition was an extraordinary endeavour, and the results lived up to its high Victorian ambition. More than 4,000 previously unknown species were discovered, some of which are still being studied today. The building's hidden history suited it. It spoke of our long, heroic and often rapacious obsession with unravelling the mysteries of life and death. With diving deep, and facing death.

On foot, I had to walk up a vertiginous hill to get there, which meant arriving with my heart kicking at my breast, making me feel as appallingly flushed with life as you could be when entering a place where people go to die. I feared walking in there, hearing the doors shoosh closed behind me, sealing normal life out. Yet once I was in it was not such a fearful place. Entering a hospice was like being let in on a secret. There was a certain amount of privilege involved in being permitted early entry to a club to which, eventually, we would all belong. It had the power to level and soothe, like the calm one enjoys walking through a graveyard, reading strangers' headstones and feeling a secondary sadness that is not so different from an appreciation of life.

I imagined a hospice would be a much more tranquil place than a labour ward, where the fight for life was paramount, and the pain of birth was expected, vital and necessary. Silence prospered in a hospice. People spoke with eyes and hands because words had no use. The smallest of gestures swelled with grandeur. The fivers in the donations box. The can of

Guinness we split between four plastic cups to make one last
toast. The most mundane of objects became suffused with a
meaning that did not belong to them. It was the strangest
kind of anthropomorphising – things took on the qualities
not of people but of feelings. Perhaps it was the absurd fact
that these beds, pens, loose change, pay-per-use TVs and
the bunch of secondhand books for sale in the café would
outlast the people dying in their midst. So they began to
absorb the grief around them. A wooden chair in an oblong
of pale northern sunlight sighed with death's loneliness. An
old man's clothes in a plastic bag hanging by his bedside were
a favourite joke well told.

Sometimes death felt like a disease you could catch and I
would wash my hands over and over again when I got home.
Yet there were so many tiny moments, each one a greatest
hit, a savage blow, and a lure designed to reel one back in to
the warmth of life. Each one pinned to memory with the terrible sweetness of being among the last ones. Like the palliative nurse who took the trouble to knock on Andy's window
one evening to wave goodbye before she cycled away, and
the way he smiled at her, just as he had smiled at us from
all those pub windows. Maybe she made a point of saying
goodbye to everyone, every night, knowing as only someone in her position could that each of those bright, cheerful
waves had the potential to be the last goodbye.

Or like how Andy asked Claire to load up her iPod with
Willie Nelson albums and then sat with this unfathomable
twenty-first-century gadget in his shaky hands, turning the
glossy dial with a finger he kept wetting with his tongue,
as though it was a book and he was a man whiling away an
afternoon in a public library with his glasses perched on the
bridge of his nose.

Expecting

Death could crush a strong man between finger and thumb, begin the business of rubbing him out even as he lived. It could return him to the childhood he had spent a lifetime growing out of, escaping, papering over. It could make him need those first simple comforts again: a song, a story, someone to pat you to sleep in the night. And pregnancy could turn the clock back too. In some ways, the more I grew, the more I felt like a child: someone who needed looking after and protecting from the world. I wanted to take in only positive information. The ten o'clock news could make me shed tears. I stopped reading newspapers. I could watch only films with happy endings. I could read only fiction. Again, the euphemistic language of pregnancy veiled a partial truth. I really did feel in a delicate condition.

Another memory, much earlier, of my mother returning from India after her mother had died. She had gone home (because that's what my parents inexplicably called this foreign land) for the funeral. My father, sister and I went to meet her at the airport. I remember feeling awkward, sullen and frightened. And then out of arrivals she came, weeping openly as soon as she saw us. My memory of all this is hazy – which airport? How old was I? Did we embrace? What words were spoken? – and yet I can summon her expression as clearly as I can bring my own palm in front of my face. Eyes wide, flitting about, impulsive. Mouth set in open, unstoppable anguish. She looked young, reckless, like she might not stop for us. I remember thinking I ought to feel something. I remember feeling nothing. Grief, on top of a spell in an unknown motherland, had rearranged her features. Made her look like a stranger to her own daughter.

And then it happened, a few days before my birthday. Or rather my Birth Day, as I was starting to think of it, cracking the word in half as Margaret Atwood does in *The Handmaid's Tale*, revealing its contents for the first time: the knowledge that my birthday was not only the day on which I was born, it was the day my mother gave birth to me. I started to feel a series of quickenings in my uterus. I say a series, because they felt multiple. This was no defined kick, tap, flutter, hunger pang or bubble of gas. It didn't remotely fit with the image of a woman pressing a hand to her bump in shock that I had seen in countless films and television series over the years. I was in no particular place when it happened, and there was no outward recognition when it did. I wasn't even sure if it was what I thought it was at first. And yet, something electrical, like the fusing of wires. A string of lights flickering, then turning on. Swaying. Soft knock-knock against the wall of my womb. Shadows in an old cave. Each time I felt these sensations, I felt jubilant, proud, as if my body had made a clever discovery and was exclaiming, 'Ah-ha!' Each one was a yes resounding through my body, the most literal affirmation of life. Of the foetus, yes, but I didn't expect its stirrings to revitalise my own sense of being here, in this moment and time, full of my own too-quick life.

I thought of those early movements as the Quickenings, as if they were a band of independent creatures bombing against my womb, rubbing feathery backs across its arches as they scuttled back and forth, stomping tiny feet across spongy surfaces. They were so different in sensation, mood, character and appearance. One day, a shoal of minnows, flipping, floundering and chasing one another's tails in a deep thrashing pool. The next, moths beating papery wings against dehydrated insides that were ribbed like the roof of a mouth. Big wet bubbles rising in mirth. No, cool smooth pebbles drifting to the bottom of a pond, tracked by quivers of sunlight. They were stars shooting in an amniotic firmament. Popcorn puffing up in a microwave. Piano scales. An army of ants tickling my insides with an enormous ostrich feather. I recalled the poet Kate Clanchy's description of her baby's first movements feeling like '... an eager, even over-familiar, / uncle-ish hard tweak at my waist'. There really was something cheeky about it. These Quickenings had personality. It was like the foetus knew me more than I did him. On a number of occasions I actually laughed out loud at the absurdity of this naughty-limbed creature. The most private of jokes.

There is a sound that icebergs make as they drift across Arctic oceans. Though one imagines nature's sculptures to be silent, ice is no less noisy and irrepressible than its liquid cousin. The song of the iceberg is a deep snap and crackle, the sound of its insides melting, bubbling, being pummelled and ripped asunder by the very substance that makes it. The sound of a cube of ice popping in a glass of lemonade, writ large. To me, it became the overriding metaphor of quickening. I felt big and glassy like an iceberg, with all the combined strength and fragility that comes with being made of a solid substance that can melt away to nothing.

The most surprising part of all this was how unsurprising it felt. My more squeamish, pre-pregnant self had imagined feeling a baby's movements as alien, possibly even disturbing. A jumble of elbows and toes doing their own thing in your body. How could it be otherwise? But the opposite turned out to be true. They were reassuring, sweet, lovable. To feel their absence was to pine for them. To feel them return was to sigh with relief. Each one was an exhibit A to be zipped up in a clear bag and treasured. Not that there was any keeping hold of them. They were as slippery as fish. Each one cancelled out the last, just as my footprints were being rubbed out as I continued through my pregnancy. The pregnant body was fickle like that, always fussing over its current state. Quickening was the most extraordinary and literal way of a body marking its present moment, a womb-print all of its own.

Leo Tolstoy astutely understood quickening's existential stamp on a woman's body, despite obviously never having felt it himself. Not surprising, perhaps, for a writer so attuned to the condition of being alive that he was even able, in his masterpiece *Anna Karenina*, to enter the mind of a dog. His great novel contains a scene in which Anna and her lover Vronsky are having another of their agonising discussions about the doomed future of their affair. Anna is pregnant with Vronsky's baby and tells him of a terrible dream in which she foresees her death in childbirth. Vronsky attempts to comfort her, but privately he too fears calamity. It is a moment of high passion and a brutal exposition of the unspoken terror that hovers above two people desperately in love. However, right in the middle of this, Tolstoy reminds us that they are no longer only two people: 'But suddenly she stopped. The expression on her face changed instantly. Terror and anxiety suddenly gave way to an expression of quiet, serious and blissful attention. [Vronsky] could not understand the meaning of this change. She had felt the stirring of new life inside her.' And just like that, the chapter ends.

The Quickenings continued, and I continued to be mired in thoughts of death. I felt removed from myself as one does when experiencing grief. I started to feel the need to leave my own body, to watch things unfold from another place. I remembered this feeling from my childhood, when I would tell myself the story of my life as I was going about living it, both for my own amusement and because I couldn't help it, but also, I wonder, to protect myself from it. I also remembered the feeling of detachment from seeing Andy in the weeks leading up to his death. I developed the capacity to remove myself when visiting him at the hospice. To look at the photos of his grandchildren pinned haphazardly to a cork board. To talk to him about the craftsmanship of the wooden chairs in a room of the hospice called The Sanctuary, to sit with him at the window of that otherwise empty room, looking out at the world that continued to turn on its axis beyond the walls of that still place. The detachment wasn't unpleasant either. It felt necessary. The philosopher David Hume writes about this removal in an autobiography he penned in a single day in 1776 not long after learning he was terminally ill. 'It is difficult to be more detached from life than I am at present,' he writes in the midst of what he terms his 'speedy dissolution'. And yet, he goes on, 'were I to name a period of my life, which I should most choose to pass over again, I might be tempted to point to this later period'. Dying, it turned out, could be a flowering too.

On my birthday we went to a hip restaurant in an old timber yard with a couple of friends. The menu was made up of small plates of bold, clever food, much of it served raw, smoked, pickled, barely cooked, strewn with edible flowers and so on. It would have thrilled my non-pregnant self, but that day I felt as unadventurous as a teenager. I sat sipping champagne that tasted more like cider, pretending to follow the conversation while the baby fizzed in my belly. I said nothing about this furtive firework display. I had no desire to talk about it. There was nothing for anyone else to feel, nothing for anyone else to understand. This was my secret Morse code tapping out its message on my insides. I felt flushed with joy. It was one of the happiest moments of my life, one I can summon up whenever I want to, and often do. And like all of the greatest instances of happiness, it passed quietly, inarticulately, uneventfully, noticed by no one but myself.

It was not unlike the wild moments of grief I saw Claire experience and felt something of myself in the weeks leading up to and just after Andy's death. Raw, reckless and utterly unreasonable, it was the feeling inspired by bearing witness to death – or, I was starting to realise, birth – in all its mad extremity. 'She began to wish she had not come; her presence was not necessary,' Kate Chopin writes of her heroine Edna Pontellier as she watches her friend give birth in the closing chapters of *The Awakening*. 'She might have invented a pre-text for staying away; she might even invent a pretext now for going. But Edna did not go. With an inward agony, with a flaming, outspoken revolt against the ways of Nature, she witnessed the scene of torture.'

Here was the extreme sport of emotion. Witnessing death, and birth, could make you race down a hill on your bike, eyes watering, hands hovering over but never coming down on your brakes. It could make you stop your car on a hard shoulder to rage at life's cold indifference even while the rest of the world speeding past on the motorway, oblivious and cocooned as babes in wombs, reassured you to your core. It could make you walk out of a hospice with the icy wind whipping off the Forth seizing your throat, and feel senselessly and gratefully alive. Or it could make you sit quietly in a restaurant that centuries ago stored props and costumes crafted by fingers crafted in utero, with your hand on your own industrious belly, feeling more present than you ever thought possible.

Which brought me back to *Anna Karenina*. After many earlier attempts I finally read this novel when I was pregnant, not realising until I arrived at it, that it contains perhaps the greatest, certainly the most detailed, scene of childbirth in fiction. It was so vivid it frightened me. I was not ready to read it, but there it was. The birth of Kitty's baby, coming towards the end of the novel, witnessed entirely through the eyes of her devoted husband, Levin, a character based on Tolstoy himself. It is a remarkably emotional scene, even in a novel renowned for its supreme commitment to the emotional truth of its characters, no matter how contradictory and inexplicable. One critic described Tolstoy as 'a slave to truth' and nowhere is this more apparent than in Kitty's labour. Watching her 'sufferings' unfold over 22 hours is a transformative experience for Levin, just as watching his brother Nikolai die a year earlier turned out to be. Levin understands that the outcomes of birth and death are diametrically opposed. One results in presence, the other absence. One induces a crisis in his faith, the other restores it. And yet his response to birth and death is overwhelmingly the same.

'He knew and felt only that what was being accomplished was similar to what had been accomplished a year ago in a hotel in a provincial capital, on the deathbed of his brother Nikolai. But that had been grief and this was joy. But that grief and this joy were equally outside all ordinary circumstances of life, were like holes in this ordinary life, through which

something higher showed. And just as painful, as torment-
ing in its coming, was what was now being accomplished;
and just as inconceivably, in contemplating this higher thing,
the soul rose to such heights as it had never known before,
where reason was no longer able to overtake it.'

Six

April

For being a foreigner ... is a sort of lifelong pregnancy – a perpetual wait, a constant burden, a continuous feeling out of sorts. It is an ongoing responsibility, a parenthesis in what had once been an ordinary life, only to discover that previous life has vanished, replaced by something more complicated and demanding. Like pregnancy, being a foreigner ... is something that elicits the same curiosity from strangers, the same combination of pity and respect.

The Namesake, Jhumpa Lahiri

The photo was taken on Claire's phone. Stored not in an attic, to be happened upon while rummaging through old shoeboxes, but on a smartphone. To be summoned up with the swoosh of a finger across mirrored black glass at any time, any place, anywhere. It was taken on a crisp, sunny day in April when I was six months pregnant. One of those days when summer, at last, seems a possibility. The location was a pub in Leith with a menu written in Scots that was supposed to be ironic and cocktails served in vintage teapots that were not. Or rather, the photo was taken outside the pub, against a dampened red sandstone wall warmed by sunlight the colour of weak tea: the backdrop of so many Scottish summers. A diagonal shadow runs just across the heads of the photo's subjects, hovering over them like a premonition. The subjects are myself and my donor.

We are both smiling the uncertain but game smiles of people thrown together in unusual circumstances. Wedding-day faces, though this was nothing like that union. Still, the look of people haunted by the ghost of sincerity: that cere-monial tightness about the mouth, expressions held a little too long, the suspicion that it's been a while since anyone has taken a breath. My arm is linked through his, a ges-ture casually intended but formal in appearance. My belly, ample now, presses lightly against his elbow. He is midway through rolling a cigarette, the paper poised between rough working-man's fingers. We do not look a likely pair, but we are trying. Our gazes are shy, directed at the photographer, Claire. The third part of our triptych, the one who is absent but present nonetheless.

I wanted this photo to be taken for the fourth person who is both in and not in the photograph. The one most unseen and to whom it belongs the most. The foetus. Made of myself and him. Belonging to myself and her. Mostly, already, just himself. Though we were now six months into our relation-ship, this limbed creature and I, though I had seen him twice on a screen and felt him jostling inside me with such idi-osyncrasy and determination that I was convinced I knew him, I still could not call him mine. Never *my baby*, always *this baby*. That baby. The baby. Sometimes, when I was feel-ing playful, *boyoboy*. Increasingly, *boyo*. This unwillingness to claim a baby rubbing up against my insides, forged from my genes and fattened on my blood, bothered me. It felt like a paucity of feeling and a foreshadowing of something dark and unnameable that I suppose was maternal guilt. I worried about it continuing.

When I told people, men and women, they were so quick to reassure me that it would be different when I set eyes on him, held him for the first time, felt his tiny fingers curl round mine, looked into his black beady eyes ... and so on. This readiness to whip out the stock images of afterbirth as though they were a weapon against the tyranny of genuine feelings seemed to be as much about shutting down the pregnant woman as placating her. And to some extent it worked. I did feel reassured, but only as a person in a play is relieved when her fellow actor gets his lines right. I felt a pressure to keep the dialogue flowing. The satisfaction came from giving the listener what he, rather than I, needed: to swaddle the pregnant woman in platitudes and keep her from the truth. Mostly, though, I felt as I often did when talking about my pregnancy: that there was a silence at the heart of it. We were not supposed to tell.

Meanwhile I was bowled over by the casual intimacy other pregnant women displayed when they talked about 'my baby', throwing their ownership of the creatures crawling about their wombs into the conversation as if it was the most obvious thing in the world. Their babies seemed to belong to them so unequivocally, so easily. Sometimes I wondered whether my inability to feel the same boiled down to the way this particular baby was conceived. With a stranger, not a lover. A man, not a father. Was I afraid of not being able to love the baby because of this? Did it weaken our sense of belonging to one another? My rational, social, political and feminist self fiercely resisted this interpretation but my emotional self, the one in charge on this particular journey, was a flighty creature upon whose soft mound of flesh opinions could be easily impressed. Society seemed to know this and tattoo its sermon on her ever more indelibly. The pregnant woman was governed by something even more unruly than her emotions: her hormones. There was no controlling these endlessly reproducing concoctions that ricocheted around my body with such fierce intent. I was vulnerable even to myself. And sometimes, most bewilderingly of all, my pregnancy made me conventional. I found myself wanting to fit in for the first time in my life, to talk about *my* baby, to be like other pregnant women.

And so the questions kept coming. Was the gulf between myself and the baby, which seemed separated by so much more than skin, blood and womb-wall, compounded by the fact that he was male? Might I have felt differently if I was carrying a girl? Would it affect my ability to birth him? Would it really change when I saw him? What would I say to all the people who peered in the buggy and asked if he looked like his father? How would I know when he did look like his father, a face with whom I was so little acquainted? Sometimes the baby seemed more of him than me. Sometimes I felt like a surrogate for myself, a tortoise with another creature's shell on its back, destined to be a stranger to everyone involved.

On the other hand, something remarkable, even familial, happened when I looked at this photograph. As soon as it was taken, even as the little button with its little haptic click was pushed, I found myself unable to look at it with my own eyes. I could not see it as myself. Every time I looked at it, which wasn't often, I could see it only through the eyes of the boy inside me. It happened instantaneously. There I was, years down the line, inhabiting this shadowy boy-man who didn't even exist yet, but who suddenly was here, behind my eyes, looking at an old photo of his mother and the man who made him. The father, as he might call him. The boy-man is intrigued. He cannot stop looking for traces of himself in both faces. Even when he doesn't look, he can still see the figures standing side by side. The photo has been stored in the attic of his mind. He no longer needs to see it to see it. The belly pressed against the elbow. The game expressions. The warm terracotta of the pocked stone: Mediterranean in colour, Scottish in character. The shape of the man's hands rolling a cigarette. He looks at his own hands. He feels lost and invisible, as we tend to when confronted by photos of our parents in that curiously empty before-time when we were not yet in the picture. He does not understand how any of it happened.

Seeing that photo was, in retrospect, my first experience of motherhood. It was the first time I experienced seeing the world twice: simultaneously through my own and my child's eyes. It was the first time I absorbed his viewpoint, or rather my perception of his viewpoint, with neither will nor intention, fusing them somewhere womb-like so that I could no longer tell them apart. This rich double take on the world was, in fact, motherhood as it is experienced every day in a million unspoken ways. I had no idea, not yet, that I would give birth to a new person and a new perspective: a dividing of self that would end up being a duplication. 'Every moment happens twice,' writes Zadie Smith in her first novel, *White Teeth*. 'Inside and outside, and they are two different histories.' How funny that this particular form of double vision started when one of us remained inside the other, his history still unmade.

I recall other moments that took place that day, ones that were not captured by any lens but which seem frozen in time nonetheless. It's as though they are photographs too: composed, framed, a little self-conscious. Here is one: we are sitting at a table in the pub, eating burgers. Claire and I are opposite our donor, our heads tilted as we watch him lift a trouser leg to reveal a sturdy man-shin, made for walking and squatting down to explain things at ground level. You cannot see my face but if you could you would think I was amused. Then, if you looked again, you would realise that it isn't amusement after all, but shock.

In that moment we were wondering about the potential skin colour of the baby, as all those with mixed-race children surely do at some point. Our donor, who is white, lifted his trouser leg to show us the colour of his skin. It was pale and softly freckled, the lightest eggshell in the box. I was shocked by the simple fact that this baby in me, the one who I couldn't yet call mine, was made of a man whose legs I had never seen. I don't recall saying anything. I may have gawped like a child. I probably giggled, as I have a tendency to do in situations that aren't exactly funny. Meanwhile, as I care-fully chewed down small mouthfuls of burger so as not to activate the dreaded heartburn, the foetus tub-thumped my belly in drunken jubilation. Little toothless carnivore, high on red meat. It seemed feasible that he was listening in on our conversation, wondering what the hell was going on, just as I imagined the people at the next table were doing. All of them thinking: what brings these people together? One dark, two light. Two women, one man. One pregnant. What could they possibly have in common? The answer, of course, was nothing and everything.

After all, the baby could hear now. And his eyes were open, blinking and capable of focusing. He could sense changes in light through all those subterranean layers of womb, muscle, fat and skin, like the mole who knows from deep in his underground burrow when the sun has gone down. He was swallowing vast quantities of amniotic fluid, the reverse of a fish rising to the surface of the water to gulp air. My placenta was working hard, a busy processing facility disposing of the waste passed along the umbilical cord back into my blood. I was carrying almost a pint of amniotic fluid now, a pool from a children's fable that magically refilled itself every three hours.

Most clearly, the foetus had his own rhythms. The 7am jig that roused me faster than any alarm clock. The long afternoon sleeps during which I waited giddily for him to wake as I had once waited for lovers to text me back. Fisticuffs on the sofa in the evening. And the best quickening drama of all was in the bath, where my belly rose out of the steam like some magnificent desert island, the surface of my skin rippled and rolled like water, and the baby paddled in his own amniotic sea. I couldn't take my eyes off the show.

Of course I could play Mozart to the baby if I chose, but life's soundtrack was invariably harsher and less composed. The world seemed shockingly loud. Vulgar, almost. My overwhelming response to so much of it – a car on the road, a person walking behind me, an ad break on television, a row on BBC Radio 4's *Today Programme* – was 'Get away from us.' I watched *Vertigo* and its male voyeurism and obsessiveness made my skin crawl. I felt dizzy when I heard Bernard Hermann's sublime vertiginous score, as though I was the foetus listening to it for the first time, panicked by its swirling dissonance. I saw Quentin Tarantino's *Django Unchained* in the cinema and spent the entire film with my hands wrapped around my belly, the pregnant woman's equivalent of covering her ears. Guns fired, slaves were beaten, everyone cursed, the foetus drop-kicked in protest and I felt stupidly, unbearably guilty. We were experiencing life side by side and I was responding to its everyday excesses as if I, not he, were the foetus, sensing it all for the first time without the protection of a womb-shield. Though he was the one imprisoned in a body, it was I who felt claustrophobic. Stuck inside my stretching, itching skin and my pregnancy. There was still such a long way to go. The hardest part was yet to come. I could feel the space in my body running out, the organs forced to rearrange themselves like children in a school year photograph. My breath was shortened daily by my ballooning uterus as it pushed ever harder on my rib cage. Sometimes it felt as though the baby was pressing the tiny heels of his hands against my ribs, gently prising them apart.

Another generation, another photo. One I have seen only a handful of times in my life, the last being many years ago. And yet, like this other photo, this latest branch of the family tree not yet ready to bud, I do not need to hold it in my hand to have it before my eyes. It is of my father before I was born. The shot black and white, small and square. Grainy in the way the world is if you half-close your eyes and let life swim into an unthreatening haze. My father – skinny Indian, cheeky chap, city slicker – is standing in the centre of the photograph, looking right at the viewer. He is wearing a shirt, flared trousers, sideburns and a cavalier expression. He is cool, streetsmart, handsome. He looks like Yul Brynner in *The King and I*, at least to me, his daughter, charmed and possibly deluded. There is no recognisable background that I can recall, merely a length of bleached street, yet I know. This is London in the Sixties. My father, born four years before India gained independence, has recently arrived from Bangalore. It is October 1967, a matter of months after what will come to be remembered, however falsely, as the Summer of Love. My father is part of the massive influx of immigrants from former colonies that took place during the Fifties and Sixties and transformed Britain forever. But change has not come yet. Carnaby Street may be experiencing a sexual revolution and the economy may be desperately in need of people like my father, but the BBC is still screening *The Black and White Minstrel Show*. The Race Relations Act has been in force for only a year, before which it was still legal to deny housing or employment based on race, nationality or ethnicity. My father, just like every other person imprisoned in their times, knows nothing of all this. He touches down at Heathrow Airport, alone, excited, skint and determined to stay.

All my father has on his person are a few clothes and a towel that I will chide him for still using decades down the line. He is allowed to bring only three pounds and twelve shillings into the country, a limit set by the Indian authorities. One of my mother's classmates – though my father and mother have not yet met – meets him at the airport. He brings him forty pounds, which my father has saved in rupees and given to this man's parents in India to send ahead of him, the way wealthy Brits used to send on their luggage before going on holiday. Forty pounds is a lot of money, not much less than the average monthly wage. This man tells my father the YMCA charges seven pounds a week and the money will last him while he looks for work. Then he leaves.

In just a fortnight my father blows his carefully saved forty pounds on trips to the theatre to see Chaucer's *Canterbury Tales*. On Paul Schofield in TS Eliot's *The Cocktail Party*, or was it *A Man for All Seasons?* He can't quite remember. Anyway, there are dinners, drinks and long walks home from Kensington and Soho in the English winter, which he recalls as being particularly harsh. He embraces this arrogant imperial city thrumming with warped reminders of home wholeheartedly, knowingly, hook, line and sinker. I love this story: its Englishness filtered through colonised, ironised eyes. I love its immigrant's defiance, openness, recklessness and pride. Was he homesick? He says not. Was he having a ball? Not exactly. He was looking for work.

In the evenings, he heads home to Hampstead Heath, a brown-skinned Dickens nightwalking the city, nothing since that morning's chapatis and curry in his belly. His address is 1 Parliament Hill, a magnificent townhouse run by a Maharashtrian cook from the YMCA called Gulhani, who puts up thirty-six Indians in its divided rooms. Every time a letter arrives addressed to my father it emboldens him to stay. He has the right: historically and presently. Look, here is the letter to prove it. He tells a story, in fact, about a letter from the mother of one of his housemates sent to 1 Parliament Street, London, by mistake. Not the lodgings of her immigrant son but the offices of Parliament. The crossed-out stamps and marks on the envelope trace its three-month journey across the capital, from Whitehall to various streets beginning with Parliament, then the post office distribution centre, and finally to the house with all the Indians in Hampstead Heath. A very British story, as my father puts it with one of his gigantic, nicotine-stained laughs. The point is, it got there in the end. All this and so much more I get from looking at this photo. Or rather not looking at it, but seeing it nonetheless.

I don't know who took it. In fact, I realise as I write this that I have never even considered this question before. It's as though it emerged out of the glossy black all by itself. A moment in time captured by some invisible, omniscient narrator of our story. Or sometimes I feel as though I took it myself, as though my father is looking at me, his future daughter, one of many lines that will anchor him to this cold country. Sometimes the two photos merge into one, though one is in colour and the other black and white, one on a phone and the other out there in the world, one of the present and the other of the past, one of two people and the other of one. When I look at them in the dark room of my mind, they start to seep into one another in the same way our dreams do with waking life. The same massive noses common to my father's side of the family. The same out-siderness, imposed but also accepted. The same proud and determined expressions. The same people.

I was thinking more of the baby now, which in turn made me think more about birthing him. This was becoming more of a reality, though the onslaught of labour remained elastic. Sometimes it was a lifetime away, like the hill that is a mere blip on the horizon. On other mornings it was the peak towering in front of me. As I approached my third trimes-ter I was gaining a warped perspective of my birth as one's view is distorted on a walk. When granted vast amounts of room to see, with horizons shimmering at the limit of our gaze, the eye no longer perceives the land in its correct order. What is very faraway can seem closer, more detailed, more real even, than what is right in front of us. The peak becomes more tangible than the path. I distinctly remember noticing this unstable and dream-like way of seeing in the ancient landscape of Assynt in the north-west Highlands. A place where the mountains seem to have names from undiscovered Norse myths – Suilven, Canisp, Quinag – and the rocks are among the oldest in the world. And when the land's skeleton is laid bare in the same way that pregnancy lays the body bare it does weird things to your eyes. The bogland stretching out from my feet seemed remote and out of focus, though I was standing in it, the toes of my boots puddled into its mulch. A loch a couple of hundred yards ahead was a mirage in the basin of the glen. The further my eyes travelled, the more real the landscape became. I felt I could reach out and touch the pink Torridon sandstone of hills that were miles away, feel their smooth surface cracked like old leather against my cold hand. The water running down the sides of the hills, trickling through ancient scree that glinted like snow, made me thirsty. I felt its cool mineral taste at the back of my mouth. The ridge of a mountain was forbidding yet oddly accessible to my mind. It was as though I could feel its porcupine spikes of rock beneath my boots. Perhaps this is what Nan Shepherd meant when she wrote that walking made her feel as if her eyes were in her feet. This was pregnancy's effect too: an enriching kind of confusion. A temporary synaesthesia of mind and body. My perspective was all over the place.

There were now moments when I felt genuinely excited at the thought of childbirth. I wanted to see myself in labour, to know this hidden part of myself. I wanted to meet this latent madwoman who had been carefully obscured by my socially acceptable self over a lifetime. By the person who signed off emails, inserted tampons and picked up her dog's shit every day with a black bag. All the stuff that fills up our lives, sets us apart and distracts us from the fact that we're basically animals who stood up too fast. I wanted to watch her wake up, rise to the occasion and howl in the face of unspeakable pain. I wanted to hear the sounds she would make, see the faces she would pull and feel how her body would command her into positions unknown. I wanted to experience the sensation of knowing what to do when no one else did.

Expecting

I was more or less decided on a home birth. I had no fear of hospital beyond the normal dread, but there was something so appealing about being in my own home, surrounded by my things, sitting on my toilet, closing my shutters and writhing on my floor. A home birth solved the problem of when to go to hospital: the concerns about getting there too early and being sent home or getting there too late and giving birth in the car park. I liked the thought of not going anywhere. Pregnancy had turned me into a homebody. And then there was the magical time after the birth, when the three of us, four including the dog, would lie in our own bed, exhausted and blown away. A family. That soft-focus bewitching hour brimming with love, hushed voices and tiny things – vests, muslin squares, feet – otherwise known as the birth of motherhood. But it was still difficult to access this place. I was always watching it through veiled curtains.

Nevertheless, I was finally beginning to think about pregnancy's afterlife. So far this experience had been an end in itself, a journey undertaken for the hardship, character-building and views from the top. For the having done it as much as the doing of it. That there would be a baby at the end of it all had never properly occurred to me, which sounds ridiculous when there is clearly no other point of pregnancy. Yet it had taken six months of gestation for this idea to properly form. Not exactly that I was going to be a mother, more that there was going to be a baby. The two things seemed separate. I struggled to understand the logic that one depended on the other for its existence.

I told Sarah, my midwife, that we were thinking about a home birth and she was delighted. No fear or hesitation. If she had concerns she didn't voice them to me. This was so different from how others responded. I began to dread telling people and when I did, my fear was often well founded. Why take the risk? Why tempt fate with a first birth? What if something went wrong? What if I couldn't cope with the pain? What if there were complications? What about the baby? The questions, at some level, were sensible and right. They came from the modern world of hospital targets, best possible outcomes and the bright lights of the operating theatre. The world in which I lived. The problem was that this was not the world of labour, which I sensed happened somewhere else where nothing could be foreseen. It was the inside of the mountain. The black hole where animals went to birth and die. So I couldn't listen to them. If I let doubt in I would never be able to banish it. My labour would be contaminated by adrenaline and fear.

I discussed my birth plan at one of my routine midwife appointments, which were now so familiar I was like a child with a sticker, pleased as punch with my proficiency at all the little medical rituals. Easing myself onto the bed to get my bump measured, which was achieved with a tape measure of all things. How reassuring to feel the old-school pressure of its end against the top of my pubic bone and then watch Sarah track an arc over my belly to the top of my abdomen, drawing me up as if I were a length of fabric. Pregnancy was meticulous work, as precise as a dress pattern, and my bump always measured within a centimetre or so of the number of weeks I was pregnant. Sometimes it was spot on: the body marking space and time in perfect synchronicity. Then my blood pressure, the urine sample and the listen-in to the baby's heartbeat. Always, it hammered, strong and fast, though it had continued to slow week on week as he lived his little life in miniature. On one visit it mimicked the cantering of hooves, on another the thunder of an express train. 'Ah,' said Sarah, 'when it sounds like a train it means you're having a boy.' We looked at each other and smiled.

After all, a home birth, for so many women over so many generations, is just a birth. There is no need for a separate classification: it is simply how it is done. Squatting and cursing among your own pots and pans. Lying in bed afterwards, a glistening baby in your arms and blood on your sheets. Would those banal still lives in all our homes – the stuffed glass cabinet, toothbrushes kissing in their little holder, one's own sweet bed – ever look the same? Or would you forget what your possessions had witnessed and continue to live among them, just as you had before.

One does not have to go far back in one's own history to find a baby born at home. My mother entered the world in the same house in which her mother was born. Like most people, she knows virtually nothing about her birth. I asked her and my father, each in their seventies, about their births and not only did I discover that both had a grandmother who had died in childbirth, but that they hadn't known this about each other, despite being married for almost forty years. In fact, it was clear that neither of them had spoken about their births before. And why would they? It is a curious fact of life that our births remain as unavailable to us as our deaths. There may be people we can ask, but we do not. Perhaps we prefer not to know. Perhaps the silencing of pregnancy and labour is so engulfing, it is passed on to the child at the moment of birth. The pact is drawn up: the one who was born will never ask and the one who birthed will never tell. Or perhaps we do not understand our gestations and births as events at all.

Until I became pregnant I was merely born, like David Copperfield in the first line of Dickens's most autobiographical

novel, though not as he was 'with a caul, which was adver-
tised for sale, in the newspapers, at the low price of fifteen
guineas'. (A caul being an unbroken amniotic sac, a rarity in
childbirth and in some cultures seen as a sign of good luck.)
What happened in the hours, days and nine months prior
to the moment of my birth became of interest only when I
became pregnant. The first line of our life stories tends to
begin after we are born. We can no more write our prologues
than our epilogues.

These are the bare facts of my mother's birth, out of which
a story must be fleshed. She was born in Bangalore in Sep-
tember 1943. The monsoon month. Four years before independence. Two years before the end of the Second World
War. She was born in a time that must have felt like the eye
of the storm but was actually approaching its end. Her parents lived in a village established in the 1880s as a colonial
settlement of quaint village greens and Mangalorean tiled
bungalows called Whitefield, where her father was a doctor.
Whitefield is now, in the way so many tales of globalisation
go, a beacon of the Silicon city. An uber-modern district of
steel, glass, high-rises, it is home to Bangalore's biggest tech
park, housing multinational giants including Xerox, IBM
and Vodafone. A whitefield still, you might say, and perhaps
of a not-so-very-different kind when you think about it.

My maternal grandfather, a doctor in his early twenties,
married my maternal grandmother when she was fifteen
years old. It took seven years for their first baby, my mother,
to arrive. She was a longed-for child, like the boy fattening
in my belly two generations down the line, across a continent, conceived under circumstances as different as it is possible to conceive. In the seventh month of her pregnancy,
my grandmother moved into her mother's house, as was

and often still is the tradition in India. An auspicious day would have been chosen and my grandmother would have been presented with a green sari by her female elders. The house was in Basavanagudi, one of Bangalore's oldest areas, named after its famous temple dedicated to the Nandi bull. My mother does not know in which room of the house she was born, but a midwife attended the birth, she believes it was 'uneventful' and she was considered to be a small baby. A cradle ceremony would have been performed after she was born in which my mother would have been placed in a cot for the first time. Months after she told me this rather spare story she sent me a follow-up email that concluded: 'Because I was in England I had none of this done for me. I am sorry I did not do anything for my girls.'

She does recall visiting the house as a child, that it was large, and that there was a champaka tree in the garden, a species of magnolia with large, fragrant blooms. Also bordering the path was a row of daffodils, the only ones my mother ever saw in India. She remembers her grandfather insisting no one talked as they ate. She does not once remember thinking of it as the place where she was born.

After my mother's birth they stayed in Basavanagudi for three months before returning home to Whitefield. By the time she was three they had left for Malleswaram, a bustling neighbourhood of Bangalore where my grandfather set up a private practice that soon got him into debt. He was a doctor renowned for giving medicine free of charge to everyone who saw him and he retained his habit of fee-waiving all his life. When he died and his study was cleared, his children found cheques that had never been cashed stored between the pages of his books. He had been using them as bookmarks.

Of Whitefield, my mother remembers nothing but has been told she was guarded by the family Alsatian who would allow no one but her parents to come near her. And that she was a very particular little girl, known for refusing to veer off the path by the house in case her feet got muddy. For a long time my mother was an only child. It was another seven years before her sister came along. It's strange. While I had always known that my mother was seven years older than her sister, I consumed this information as essential familial history, whittled down to the bare bones of numbers and names. I never once thought about those seven years as a period in time when my mother was the only child of her parents until I thought of her as a little girl in the shadow of an Alsation and, hearing the story of her birth more than seventy years later, a baby exiting her mother's body. And all this I found out because I asked my mother the question: where were you born?

I also asked her about my birth and though it took place thirty-six years after her own, the story was just as threadbare and, in a way, just as removed. It was like a tale of another generation. I had to keep reminding myself that the baby in question was, in fact, me. I was my mother's second child; my sister was two years old at the time. My mother remembers the pregnancy fondly, as a quiet time of walks along the Thames and long afternoon naps with my sister. They were living in a newly built terraced house in a cul de sac in Twickenham, south-west London. They had been there a year by the time my mother went into labour one evening 'close' to her due date. They were relaxed enough to eat their dinner before leaving for West Middlesex hospital in a taxi. I always felt a vague disappointment at being born in a hospital stuck out in the suburbs when my sister burst into the world in the midst of it all. London proper: zone one, University College Hospital, just off the Euston Road.

West Middlesex was established as a hospital in 1920 but originally opened as the Brentford Workhouse Infirmary in 1894. During the winter of 1940 the maternity wing was severely damaged by bombs and wasn't repaired until the Sixties. When I was born, West Middlesex still resembled an old and somewhat dilapidated Victorian hospital, though it has now been completely 'redeveloped' as a major London facility, funded by yet another Private Finance Initiative. I know this only because I have read about it. I have never been there since my birth. Anyway, it is a typical NHS history, mimicking that of the hospital more than four hundred miles north in Edinburgh where, thirty-five years later, I might end up giving birth myself.

My mother's labour was short, as is often the case with second babies. By the early hours of the following morning she was experiencing 'proper pains' as she calls them and I was born two hours later, pulled into the world with forceps. My head was showing but my mother needed help when her contractions 'fizzled out' in the final stage. She remembers the fear when things started to unravel, more people quickly appeared, and her legs were hoisted into stirrups. When I was born my mother, by now shaking with exhaustion, did not want to hold me. She recalls overhearing two Indian nurses in the room whispering that she was probably disappointed because I was a girl, which upset her greatly. She recalls my thick mop of black hair, which everyone in the delivery room commented on. She recalls feeling joy, relief and the most exquisite exhaustion. The story I associate most with my birth comes from another perspective completely. From my sister, who was almost three and also a forceps birth. Her birth was longer and harder. My mother was cut badly by a junior doctor in the last moments before my sister was born, a botched job that appalled the midwife who later examined her and meant she could not sit comfortably for weeks. My sister had a huge bump on her head from the forceps, so there was no photo taken of her in the hospital. Anyway, my father took her, three years on and bump-free, to West Middlesex and bought her a paper bag of penny sweets on the way, presumably to soothe the blow of my arrival. Black Jacks. Those rock-hard chews that stain your tongue and deliver a sucker punch of aniseed to your gums, mouth, throat and head. This is my sister's memory, probably her first, yet I have subsumed it into my own life story so that when I imagine my birth, I taste aniseed. It would not surprise me if I were to stick out my tongue in the mirror when I think about it, as children are wont to do, and find it was inked blue-black. I experience my birth at one remove, the only way I can. Would my made-up memory of it be remade when I gave birth? No more the taste of aniseed. No more the child's view of birth, witnessing only the end result, understanding nothing of the beginning and middle. Might I become my mother instead? Feel her 'proper pains'? The tug of the forceps? The weakness in her arms?

Towards the end of the month, Sarah came over to the flat to discuss the home birth in more detail. I felt nervous, as though she were an adoption assessor coming to judge our fitness for the job, which of course meant the dog instantly jumped all over her, yapping, nipping and uncovering our parental failings before the kettle had boiled. The dog had been acting peculiarly for a while now, attuned in that specifically animal way to my expanding belly. When I got up from a bench on a walk, she jumped up and sniffed the precise spot where I had been sitting, a detective on the scent of a dropped hormone. She did this every single time. I wondered what my pregnancy smelled like to her: blood-iron, salt and heat, the comforting smell of one's own body baking on the beach after a swim in the sea. Sometimes she rested her head on my belly and slept noisily, snoring, twitching and eye-rolling, her muzzle rising and falling with my breath, one ear pricked to the internal racket. The foetus reminded me of her, too. There was a particular way this other furry companion scrabbled about that imitated her habit of kicking out sharply with her hind legs when she was shifting into a relaxed position. The same territorial move that was more animal than human: strong, laconic and hare-like. The same staking out of space that doesn't strictly belong to you.

We walked around the flat talking about where I might give birth. Claire and Sarah were drawn to the bedroom, which made sense, but, without realising it, I had already imagined labouring in the sitting room. The light of our quadruple-headed red lamp that always had at least two bulbs missing, a birthing pool in the corner, shutters closed and Duncan Chisholm's *Strathglass Trilogy* playing on the stereo. I had become obsessed with this exquisite trio of fiddle albums inspired by Chisholm's homeland, a widescreen landscape around Glen Affric punctuated with salmon-rich rivers and remnants of original Caledonian pine forest. We listened to them constantly on a holiday in Orkney, the triptych of CDs revolving in the car because we didn't have any other music with us. A small act of forgetfulness that has entirely shaped the way I remember those lo w green humps rising from the North Sea, the Neolithic remains buried in them like unborn children, and the oil flare on distant Flotta branding a sienna tip on to the horizon. I cannot think of any of this without hearing Chisholm's restrained slow air playing. And three hundred miles away in Leith, moments from the harbour where boats sailed to Orkney from as early as 1790, I cannot play Chisholm without thinking of that holiday.

Whether any of this would transmute to my labour was another question, but Orkney had come to hold a particular significance. Though we did not know it at the time, it was our last holiday as a couple. A week spent on the far eastern peninsula of Deerness in an old farmhouse at its very tip. The last house, as the locals called it. To the north we could see the isles of Shapinsay, Stronsay and, on clear mornings, Sanday. North Ronaldsay, known for its hardy little sheep that graze on seaweed, was out there too if only we had the strength in our eyes to see it. We tweaked the ears of the goats in the morning who always rushed across the field to nuzzle us like the most loyal of dogs. We walked the headland, watching curlews scything the windblown grass and fulmars nesting in the cliffs. We searched for seals on the rocks below and got dizzy looking down into the great chasm of a collapsed sea cave known as a gloup. The Norse word for a blowhole that contains, in just five letters, all of that particular sea's voluptuous suck and slap. We found the ruins of a Norse chapel by climbing deep steps cut into sandstone, guided by a rusted chainlink rail slung between old nails. In the evenings we drank Highland Park, smoked roll-ups and read *King Lear* out loud. The next day the wind carried our hangovers away with the sea spray and racing banks of cloud and we did it all over again. It was a very grown-up holiday, but still, always, there was the persistent backing track of yearning. The desire, unlike any other. A need that could be fulfilled by one thing only. To be more than just the two of us. To have a baby. A fortnight after we returned from Orkney we got a dog, a traumatised stray rescued from a pound in South Wales who barked at the bookshelves, whinnied all night long and had the most marvellous black and white toenails. And a fortnight after that, with my eye taken off the ball by this neurotic little creature with such boundless love and need, I was pregnant.

Sarah talked through some potential issues. The two deep and winding flights of stairs leading up to our flat, for a start. When we bought the place, they had seemed full of character. A quintessential Edinburgh stair: crooked, damp, stubbornly inaccessible for more than a century and ripe with old stories and festering smells. Now, with ageing parents, a dog, a baby on the way and a future of buggy-lugging before us, they were a liability. Everyone who stood at the bottom of them looked at my belly then sucked their teeth in dismay. Those stairs actually kept me up at night. While the baby toiled in my belly and I lay stacked between ever more pillows to prop up my body, I pictured him slipping out of my arms and bouncing down those stairs. Over and over again, his soft limbs tumbling over worn stone. Blood and unconsciousness. How on earth would I manage?

Now it turned out they might also prove a problem during labour. If I needed to transfer to hospital in an emergency I would have to negotiate those stairs. One by one, counting contractions, gripping on to the shaky bannister. Then there was the strength of our floors – could they cope with the weight of a birthing pool? We would need to have a home birth box delivered by week thirty-five, though what it would contain I had no idea. We would need to keep the vitamin K injection for the newborn in our fridge, and the giant canisters of gas and air in our bedroom. The fire department would need to pay a visit. We would need to do so much. Then, of course, there would be a baby. And then … life. The to-do list really was never-ending.

Before Sarah left I told her we had just organised a holiday to the island of Mull with some friends. I would be thirty-four weeks pregnant when we were there and was concerned about going into labour, or even false labour, on the island. Sarah, who was from neighbouring Iona, reassured me in her usual quiet way and then instructed us to go to her favourite chocolate shop in Tobermory. She said that of course wherever people lived, no matter how remote or inaccessible, women gave birth. And Mull, as Scottish islands went, was a big one. Yet I had never considered the night-time dashes to hospital on twisting island roads, with only passing place signs to watch over you and the outlines of mountain and coast to offer solace. I had never thought about the terror of an unexpected birth in deep countryside. Of the plucky little plane with its labouring passenger carrying her own freight, nosing through turbulent air. One air ambulance service covering the Hebrides, Shetland and Orkney flew many pregnant mothers to hospital in the years between 1967 and 2006. The Britten-Norman Islander, built on the Isle of Wight in the Fifties and now stored at the National Museum of Scotland's warehouses in Granton, even became the makeshift maternity ward for twenty-two babies, including one set of twins, who were born onboard during forty years of avian dashes to the mainland.

Sarah knew plenty of women from tiny islands like Iona who moved to the mainland in the weeks running up to the birth to be closer to the maternity ward. Otherwise boats were often required in the middle of the night. Imagine it: riding your contractions on a bucking sea. I thought of the

Expecting

Maldives and that terrifying crossing, bumping over glassy swells with the little tadpole whirlpooling in my tummy. I thought of labouring not in water, as I wanted to, but on top of it, aimless and buoyant as a cork. Two flights of stairs in Leith seemed nothing in comparison.

Afterwards, I wandered around the flat rubbing my belly. I felt big and mild, like the First Voice in Sylvia Plath's radio play of excoriating honesty about pregnancy and birth, *Three Women*, who is 'as slow as the world / I am very patient, / Turning through my time, the suns and stars / Regarding me with attention.' The lamp, the drab corner of the room where the birthing pool might go, the Duncan Chisholm CDs stacked, no doubt in the wrong cases, by the stereo. They looked like props or photographs of themselves. The room had the air of a set abandoned just after a dress rehearsal. So did my body: even the baby was asleep. I thought of the following lines from the opening stanza of *Three Women*. It was first broadcast in 1962, a few months after the birth of Plath's son, Nicholas. And it was to be her only play. She died the following year.

> 'When I walk out, I am a great event.
> I do not have time to think, or even rehearse.
> What happens in me will happen without attention.
> The pheasant stands on the hill;
> He is arranging his brown feathers.
> I cannot help smiling at what it is I know.
> Leaves and petals attend me. I am ready.'

Seven

May

There are people who think that children are made in a day.
But it takes a long time, a very long time.
Huma Rojo, *All About My Mother*, Pedro Almodóvar

The 8am train from Edinburgh to London is a busy service. A commuter train almost, though shuttling between
Scotland and England seems an absurdity even in the twenty-first century. Those early-morning trains invariably filled
with workers at once fresh-faced and old, their laptops
flipped open in front of them as the length of Britain hurtles
past through windows looked through less than the ones
on their screens. For nigh on a decade as a journalist living
and working between cities hundreds of miles apart I had
been one of them; already tapping away on my laptop by the
time we departed Waverley, the headachy reek of the brakes
perfuming the carriages on approach to each station and my
stomach lurching when the train tilted on its tracks.

I knew the route so well I hardly needed to look out of
the window to see what was passing by. I knew when we
were going to charge through a station without stopping,
the train moving just fast enough to make the signs tanta-
lisingly unreadable. I knew the precise moment along the
coastline near Berwick-upon-Tweed when you could catch a
glimpse of a lone ruin perched above a rocky bay at Lamberton Skerrs, the most southerly point on Scotland's east coast.

Expecting

A stubborn shiel lodged between nations. A piece of history clinging to the cliff face, absorbed into the land over centuries until it was as much a part of the coastline as the rocks, the sea spraying them, and the sheep seemingly unaffected by the train zooming past at 125 miles per hour. It was an old salmon fishery, apparently known to locals as 'Lumburn' or 'The White Hoose' and used as an unofficial shore mark. Its insides had been eaten by the vestiges of time and sea (and, according to its Wikipedia page, fire), just as the skeletons of shells you find on beaches are jostled into softness. Every time I saw this little bothy, it was as though it was the first time. And every time I missed it, I promised I would look out for it on the return journey, as if my marking it was somehow necessary for it, or perhaps us, to exist.

After this was Newcastle and the thrill that comes from pulling into any industrial city over a mighty body of water. Then the imposing Victorian stations of Darlington and York, their red-brick arches made for restrained and overcast goodbyes. And finally, after slicing through black tunnel after ear-popping tunnel, King's Cross. Mouth of London, terminus of the east-coast line ever since it was constructed in 1852, one of the world's great stations with its pair of monumental arched train sheds like perpetually raised eyebrows, and home. The city in which I was born.

I was on the verge of ending this journey, at least for a while, if not forever in this particular way: on my own and in silent companionship with a route as marked, checked and crossed as a signature. In some ways it had ended already. Not only was I no longer on my own, I had entered my final trimester and travel was becoming less appealing by the day. Home was the only destination for me now. The world had stretched in such synchronicity with my body that I hadn't noticed it until everywhere seemed far away. Even my parents' second-floor council flat in London, which despite having left it almost twenty years ago was still my most fixed abode in the world. Pregnancy was a great deceiver: it could make the familiar strange and the cosy deeply uncomfortable. What was once home was now a bed without the carefully constructed architecture of pillows I needed to get through the night, no Claire beside me to soothe my hormonal night frights and lift the duvet for me on one of my many returns from the toilet, and always the lurking possibility of going into labour five hundred miles away. The third trimester brought with it a bucket list of sorts, albeit one to tick off before a beginning rather than an end. There were a lot of lasts. This particular journey to London was one of them.

The train was packed with enough commuters to ensure I had someone sitting next to me the whole way down. A middle-aged white man, smartly suited and smelling of the office: aftershave on stubbled skin, morning breath masked by coffee, the warm metallic scent of a computer waking up. He was constantly on his mobile phone despite his signal cutting out every few minutes. Beyond a mild irritation at his bull-headed persistence, I did not notice anything unusual about him. In fact, he inhabited the environment so well it worked like camouflage. I hardly noticed him at all.

I sat by the window, feeling sick with the motion as I always do when writing on trains and even more so with a baby bearing down on my insides like feet pressed into firm sand. He was now about 28cm long, almost the length of a classic school ruler, and weighed around three pounds. Sitting still seemed to be an invitation to dance. I would rest and he would get going. A foot in the ribs, a bounce on my bladder, and occasionally a full somersault, which felt like he was taking my belly with him as a person who rolls over in bed hogs the duvet. At least once a day he got hiccups, producing a series of rhythmic taps that reverberated through my belly as if he were a next-door neighbour doing DIY. I would place my hand over the spot where I imagined his hiccuping fish-mouth to be and feel as each bubble travelled up and away, over and over again. At any other time, when I put my hand on the place where he was digging in his heels, headbutting my ribs or mooning my womb with his skinny bottom, he would go completely still. The fish slithering away from the hook. Following him around my body like this was a word-less conversation, a small and familiar remonstrance between mother and son, a play we were acting out for no one but ourselves. And it happened when other people attempted to feel him move too. Always the flurry of movement, 'The baby is moving! Quick … here … feel…', followed by the search-ing pressure of someone else's hand guided by my own. Then stillness. An unruffled surface. A refusal to play the game.

Meanwhile, the man's incessant talking on his phone was beginning to irritate me. Eventually I started to eavesdrop. I caught the odd word. *Scan. Rare. Cancer.* Words that have the power to induce terror even when they're spoken by a stranger on a train whose face you've never seen front-on. Then came the platitudes – 'keeping busy', 'staying posi-tive', 'taking each day as it comes'. Those orderly and familiar phrases that become indispensable when something deeply disorderly and unfamiliar is happening to you. Language's survival kit, to be used with caution during pregnancy, birth, illness and death. It dawned on me. The man had just found out he had a terminal illness. This particular train to London was the place where he had decided to break his news to some of the people in his life.

Eventually the poor signal got the better of him and he gave up. We sat side by side in silence as the train passed Darlington, both of us making a bad job of pretending to work. I watched him out of the corner of my eye and felt oddly embarrassed at my belly protruding with such insistence that it was pressed into the table pulled down from the seat in front of me. It felt inappropriately abundant for the occasion. But then he pointed at it and said, 'and how are you getting on?' The 'and' was crucial. It signified that the conversation had already begun.

We talked with the peculiarly intense intimacy of strangers on a train. I had never had a conversation quite like it in a decade of ferrying myself back and forth between Scotland and England, sitting next to hundreds of people, each with his or her own briefcase, M&S sandwich selection and life story. Occasionally I would catch the eye of a fellow commuter, bond over some delay or random shared experience, say sorry when our feet knocked under a table, but that would be it. The possibility squeezed shut. As a heavily pregnant woman, the world dilated like a cervix. Pregnancy was nature's own form of slow travel. Journeys stretched out and became less focused on the end. There was no speeding them up. Sometimes this ponderous pace could breed the worst kind of claustrophobia: a feeling of being stuck in the lift of your own gravid body. Confined.

Again, the old words had their uses if we could only rescue them from their original meanings. From as early as the 1770s labour was known as confinement, a euphemism for the earlier 'childbed' (or, in Scots, 'jizzen', 'gizzen' or 'gissan'), demarcating the 'lying-in' period from the onset of labour to birth. The language used to describe childbirth was always shifting. While women are now said to deliver babies they were originally delivered of the baby. In other words, the woman was the passive object and it was the doctor or midwife who did the delivering. Confinement was an archaic term (though 'labour' wasn't much better at encompassing the experience) and now tends to refer to the period just after the birth. And though all of these words – 'confinement', 'lying-in', 'accouchement' ('to go to bed' in French), 'downlying' – were no longer in common usage, they weren't relegated as far back in the past as we imagined either. Walk south over London's Westminster Bridge towards Lambeth and you can still see the original grand frontage and sign of the General Lying-In Hospital, one of the first non-denominational maternity hospitals in Britain, which saw more than 150,000 births over 150 years and closed only in 1971. In a way, confinement suited pregnancy because it did imprison women: we were confined in our own bodies, in the panopticon of a society forever watching us, and by time's rigorous nine-month structure. Pregnancy as a kind of solitary confinement, restricting your liberty in the most immediate of ways.

On the other hand, things happened when you were trapped in an experience and couldn't get out. Hemmed in by time and freed by its confines, I saw more. Pregnancy as a magnifying glass, turning sand grains to pebbles and dust to bugs. The ruin at Lamberton Skerrs became a salmon fishery with a story and a Wikipedia page instead of a personal marker on a route. I saw lives where before I had seen only strangers. Conversations were struck up all over the place. The national grid of stories could be tapped. Slowing down meant you could see more of life, and life could see more of you. On the flip-side, this made pregnancy deeply exposing. As well as being a site of conflict and projection, I felt like a beacon for truth. It was a third stranger, the one growing in my belly, who prompted this man to talk to me. We would not have spoken otherwise.

I told him I was seven months pregnant with a boy who, I did not add, in forty years could be this very man sitting next to me. This, after all, was how he began. He told me he had recently been diagnosed with a rare form of incurable cancer that usually affected much older people. He did not know how long he had to live but because he was young the prognosis was good. This was the skewed logic of cancer: the part that made the news so unbearable, so unjust, was also the factor that might prolong your life. Bad and good news, handed to you at the same time. When my mother was diagnosed with breast cancer after a routine mammogram, so many people – myself included – felt it necessary to point out how lucky it was that she had gone for the mammogram at all. Imagine if it hadn't been detected? Imagine how much worse it could have been? And so it went on. She lost only one breast, not two. What if she had been younger? I remember thinking all of this myself, and finding it frightening and a relief at the same time. It was unlucky, yes, but it could have been so much worse. We talked about this appalling conundrum, this stranger and I, and I told him my mother was treated for breast cancer the same year I got pregnant. Illness and wellness, handed to us at the same time. He told me he had four children. Perhaps his voice broke, but I did not dare look at him. We both fell silent. He made no more calls.

So there we were, two strangers heading the same way for work but travelling in opposite directions in life. One pregnant with the start of everything, the other heavy with the end. It felt like a particularly crude collision but there it was. When we arrived at King's Cross after a long, companionable silence the man got my bag down for me. A small act of chivalry, of maintaining the status quo, that nearly broke my heart. We wished each other luck and went our separate ways.

Another train journey, one that also shuttles between two kinds of home in Pedro Almodóvar's *All About My Mother*. A film that was at the forefront of my mind, and perhaps my belly, too, for two reasons. One: the train journey has got to be one of the most powerful metaphors of birth, and rebirth, in cinema. Two: the train I was on was taking me to meet its director. This was why I had come to London. My last job before going on maternity leave was to interview Almodóvar.

The Spanish director's masterpiece is a love letter to women – and women in film – that most obviously pays homage to *All About Eve*. But beyond that it is a celebration, tragic and very funny, of the performance involved in becoming a mother. Its tone is dark, hysterical and hyper-real, just like the melodrama that is pregnancy and birth. And like pregnancy, *All About My Mother* takes place on its own plane of reality. Its truth is to be discovered in the uncharted emotional hinterland and scarred bodyscape of women. A place you don't get to visit until you get on a train and go there.

Transformation is Almodóvar's great theme: child to adult, man to woman, or woman to mother. *All About My Mother* teaches us that anyone can become a mother, or for that matter a woman, if they desire it, enact it, embody it and live it. If we cannot carry babies in our bodies we can still summon motherhood into our being through acts of will. We can mother without being mothers. We can mother without being women. We can be mothers without giving birth. We can mother without having children at all. All of this was of great comfort to me during the months and years when I was trying to conceive and come to terms with a future that might not have a baby birthed from my body in it. Also to Claire, a woman who wanted to be a mother but had no desire to carry a child of her own. Almodóvar's dedication at the end of the film makes all this explicit: 'To Bette Davis, Gena Rowlands, Romy Schneider ... To all actresses who have played actresses, to all women who act, to men who act and become women, to all people who want to become mothers. To my mother.' Many have claimed that *All About My Mother* is, in fact, All About Almodóvar.

The train journey takes place near the start of the film. Manuela, the mother of the film's title, is travelling from Madrid, where her son Esteban has just been killed, to Barcelona, where he was conceived. Esteban died in a car accident on the night of his seventeenth birthday. Manuela is going to Barcelona in search of his father, whom she met while playing Stella (a character who, it's worth adding, is pregnant during much of the play) in a production of *A Streetcar Named Desire*. But she is also looking for some surviving shred of herself, for a way to continue being a mother without her son, for a way to continue at all. In a life that has been robbed of meaning, she craves simple, forward-facing direction.

The scene itself is short, haunting and so symbolic that at the other end of *All About My Mother* we get its mirror image: the same train journey running in the opposite direction. In the first one, Manuela is on the train, her face a study of grief as fresh as spilled blood. Her voiceover informs us that seventeen years earlier she made the same journey, but in the opposite direction, from Barcelona to Madrid. 'I was running away then too, but I wasn't alone,' she says. 'I was carrying Esteban inside me.' It's a staggering line about loss located as much in the body as in the world. About the beguiling and frustrating fact that pregnancy invades your body so absolutely you can never be alone, anywhere, even looking out of the window on a train. It's a line about the supreme commitment involved in mothering a child, not just from birth to death but from whatever point you realise that you are no longer alone. That you never will be again. That the business of mothering, of being something other and perhaps more than yourself, has begun. That pregnancy is only the first manifestation of being two people.

A hypnotically long shot of a tunnel follows, its edges softened by light like bones bleached by the sun, accompanied by the plaintive opening bars of a song, 'Tajabone', by the Senegalese musician Ismael Lo. This is the birth canal that will carry Manuela back to her son's beginning. Finally the pinprick of light at the end of the tunnel opens – one might say like a cervix – and the camera ascends over Barcelona at night. The city: the place where anyone can go to be reborn. Gaudí's gothic and perennially unfinished fantasy, the Sagrada Familia, is reflected in the windows of a taxi as Manuela drives past post-Franco Barcelona's red-light district, circling its prostitutes, drag queens and transsexuals. Everything is dark, transgressive and shot through with the promise of violence, the blackest of humour and the explosive beauty of survival against the odds.

It is one of the most powerful scenes in the film, even though ostensibly it's just a journey from A to B. It evokes that visceral feeling of just being alive, going somewhere, revisiting the places where you became yourself. My sister and I used to love this thoroughly grown-up scene in the fierce way young people fixate on things they have yet to fully understand. We would rewind it over and over again, hungry for its indecipherable message. We could not sleep without putting on 'Tajabone', listening to it last thing at night, our minds drifting down that tunnel into the hot puppy sleep of teenagers. I'm not sure whether our obsession was about the music, Manuela's grief, Spain, our mother or the places she left that we barely knew, but it lasted. It remains one of the most replayed scenes in the picturehouse of my mind.

Each of *All About My Mother*'s explorations of pregnancy and birth seems to happen at the heightened level of metaphor. Not just birth but rebirth. Not just one birth canal, but two. Not just pregnancy, but the acting of it. Later, in a production of *A Streetcar Named Desire* in Barcelona, Manuela ends up playing a heavily pregnant Stella for one night only. Her performance is so convincing that as she goes into labour and is carried off the stage weeping in her husband Stanley's arms like a child we realise she is not acting at all, but grieving for her dead son. The one she was carrying seventeen years earlier.

Cinema is as awash with unrealistic representations of childbirth as it is of sex. It is virtually a subgenre of its own with its own emotional truth and bizarre rules. The woman's waters break in the most dramatic of circumstances but with the least amount of fluid. The rush to the hospital, preferably in a taxi. The labouring in bed, the woman always on her back. It ends quickly and without complications. A few red-faced pushes, cheerleader shouts of encouragement from the midwife, and swearing at the partner. Finally, the sighting of the head – if the father looks at this point, he is likely to keel over – and then the baby, mewling and pink-mouthed as a kitten, clean, wrapped in a blanket and about six weeks old. The mother fresh-faced. No sign of trauma, blood, vernix, stitches or a placenta. When one thinks of pregnancy and birth, images as stylised as studio stills invade the screen. *Look Who's Talking*, with its pink-washed opening scene of the sperm chasing the egg. *Friends*, with its hospital births so airbrushed that both hair and comic timing remain intact. *Lost*, with its stupefyingly fast natural births in the middle of an island in the middle of nowhere. And, perhaps most of all, *Gone with the Wind*.

In one of cinema's most famous birth scenes, the indefatigable heroine Scarlett O'Hara delivers her cousin Melanie's baby in the besieged city of Atlanta, the birth unfolding in tandem with the death throes of the Old South. In a gown the colour of old blood, Scarlett picks her way through rows of hundreds of wounded soldiers lying in the dirt of an open-air hospital with neither bandages nor chloroform. In search of a doctor to assist the delivery, when at last she finds one, Doctor Meade refuses to go with her. The drama of one birth cannot compete with this much death. 'Don't worry, child,' are his parting words. 'There's nothing to bringing a baby.'

This, of course, is far from true. Scarlett returns home and mercilessly beats the slavegirl Prissy when she confesses that she 'don't know nothing about birthing babies'. Then she demands a mystifying series of instruments – boiled water, a ball of twine, clean towels and scissors – that seemed to spawn an entire generation of birth scenes in which someone is sent off to get hot water and towels. She grips the banister, grits her teeth and heads for Melanie's bedside. Over many hours Melanie weakens, her labour pains grow, the night gets darker and hotter, and war closes in on Atlanta. Apparently Olivia de Havilland (Melanie), who had never given birth, wanted to portray the scene as realistically as possible and visited Los Angeles Hospital disguised as a nurse to observe women in labour. During filming, George Cukor, who directed the scene, twisted de Havilland's ankle or pinched her toes every time he wanted her to simulate a contraction.

It's probably Prissy who delivers the most memorable line, though, revealing that she does know something about birthing babies after all when she says her mother told her, 'if you put a knife under the bed, it cuts the pain in two'. And it is in this scene that Scarlett, among cinema's most spoilt, spiteful heroines, is at her most impressive and humane. 'Don't try to be brave, Melly,' she hisses. 'Yell all you want to. There's nobody to hear.' By the end of the night, the relationship between these two rival women is changed for life.

I met Almodóvar in the library of the Soho Hotel, where many of London's press junkets take place. I had been allotted an hour with him, an unusually generous amount of time with anyone in the industry, let alone the most successful director of non-English-language films in the world. Almodóvar insisted on doing only a small handful of interviews each day, which was a nightmare for publicists but a joy for those of us asking the questions. It gave the interview the freedom to roam. There was the sense, even before you walked into the room, that you could ask Almodóvar anything.

He looked boyishly handsome at 63 with a shock of grey hair, skin as brown as a chestnut, a generous paunch, and one of those face-consuming smiles. He had a big meaty handshake and liked to throw his pudgy hands around as he talked, stirring the air with his solid body and elegant speech. He was dressed in grey trousers and polo shirt, the requisite props of Ray-Bans and smartphone placed on the table in front of him. His eyes, which were warm, brown and commanding, briefly flickered south to my belly after we said hello. A silent acknowledgment of what lay between us. A person, but also a theme, image and metaphor that had haunted his entire body of work.

Expecting

We were there to talk about his latest film, but what we ended up talking about most was mothers. 'I could write a million stories where the mother is central,' he announced, and again his eyes lowered to my belly as if one of the scripts might be writing itself there. 'The strength of them, the way they forge ahead and get things done even in the most difficult and uncompromising of circumstances ... these are key concepts in all my films and will continue to be so.'

He spoke about his mother, the centre of his world, cinematic and otherwise, and a formidable woman with no education and a wicked sense of humour. An Almodóvar character waiting to be written. He told me how she came to live in Madrid with his sisters after their father died, just as Almodóvar was establishing himself as a renegade filmmaker in post-Franco Spain. For the last thirty years of her life, the same period in which Almodóvar became Spain's most celebrated director, their relationship became very intense. She was the greatest inspiration for his films, though she never watched them. 'She tried not to,' he told me. 'She wasn't interested in cinema.

'She wasn't a woman with small-town prejudices, though she lived in a small town her entire life,' he continued. 'She had a fantastic sense of humour. She was the star of the street. Watching her entertain the neighbours was an education. She had extraordinary initiative and she could make something out of nothing. She has been a direct inspiration for my films. I have lots of characters who talk like her.'

At the end of the interview, Almodóvar ignored the two publicists who had entered the room and continued to talk. 'I recognise the miracle of maternity,' he said and looked at my stomach, for longer this time. There it was again, the same uneasy feeling I had experienced on the train of being both more and less than myself to strangers. It made me feel proud, embarrassed and misunderstood all at the same time. And, in this case, as though my pregnancy was guiding the interview, just as it had initiated the encounter on the train. 'It is one of the only pure miracles we have,' Almodóvar continued. 'The mother is at the centre of all relationships: with men, women, children, society, land and reality. So in terms of filmmaking, she is the key for me. The mother is the Don Quixote of all my characters.'

Returning to Scotland, it felt like the drawbridge was being pulled up behind me when the train left Berwick-upon-Tweed. I tried to picture making the journey with the baby not in my belly but in my arms. Why was it still so difficult to imagine? Perhaps the time had come to put aside the fear that something could still go wrong. Perhaps the time had come to claim this baby as my own. To start buying things. Consuming seemed a superficial way to make the transition but maybe a Moses basket in the corner of our bedroom, sleepsuits, mitts and cellular blankets folded in the drawers, and all those little muslin squares that were apparently so crucial but remained as baffling to me in their use as the ball of twine in *Gone with the Wind*, would kickstart motherhood. Or at least enable me to picture it happening. It was time to look forward to life after birth. It was with a mixture of regret, melancholy and pure excitement that I sought out the ruin at Lamberton Skerrs along the coast as we thundered back to Edinburgh.

It was time to go for my thirty-two week scan to see if the placenta had orbited from its position partially eclipsing my cervix. By now this giant wombsponge weighed about a pound and was receiving half a litre of blood from my circulation every single minute. Claire was confident it had

budged out of the way and kept quoting statistics at me –
90 per cent of placentas move, women's wombs are overly
policed and scanned anyway – which was true but frustrating nonetheless because my pregnancy, from the inside, had
nothing whatsoever to do with statistics, ideology or even
feminism. It was too weird and hormonally governed to be
tamed into any theory or turned into a percentage. And so I
felt terrified. There was no getting better at pregnancy. One
did not improve as the months went on and the belly domed
higher. Rather, one became more invested, thin-skinned and
fragile. The balloon blown too large, increasingly on the
verge of popping.

The scan itself was murkier than the others, both on screen
and in my memory. What I experienced, primarily, was discomfort. For the first time lying on my back was almost
unbearable. The baby pressed down on my organs and arter-
ies like a hand holding my head under water, firm and menacing. I felt squished by my own body. Smothered by a few
stubborn pounds of personhood. I just wanted it to be over.

I lay there gritting my teeth, my bladder full and my body
begging to roll onto its side. Claire was quiet. The sonographer worked quickly, perhaps sensing my unhappy state.
In no time at all she said that the placenta had moved out
of the way and I could have my home birth. The relief was
so engulfing it blotted out everything after that moment.
I didn't see the placenta in its new position at the front of
my uterus, a thick cushion that could apparently dull the
impact of the baby's movements. A little padded cell. I didn't
see the baby on screen, just some moving images as suspect
and grainy as CCTV footage. I didn't ask the sonographer to
double check the baby's sex as I had intended to. I didn't ask
for a picture of my womb to take home.

Afterwards I felt dazed, lifestruck and as fragile as an egg. I felt as though time had suddenly speeded up and the last handful of sand was freefalling through the neck of the egg timer. 'I wasn't ready,' says the Third Voice in Sylvia Plath's *Three Women*, a college student who gives her baby up for adoption following an unwanted pregnancy. 'But it was too late for that. It was too late, and the face / Went on shaping itself with love, as if I was ready.' We went to a café for tea and cake, the eternal diet of pregnant women, which was beginning to bore me. I craved not my old life exactly, but at least some of its greatest hits. My lust for coffee, books, wine, train journeys, sleeping through the night, seeing my own feet, striding out into the hills with the dog running ahead of me, runny yolks, oysters, lying on my back in the grass and being the only person in my body was returning. I wasn't ready for motherhood but I was beginning to look forward to the end of pregnancy.

But how would it end? Until that moment it had been a possibility, and I now realised a reassuring one, that my body was going to make the decision for me. But the placenta had moved and the choice had been handed back to me. I could give birth naturally, whatever that meant. And no matter how it happened, this baby was coming. He would be here in eight weeks. It seemed at once like the blink of an eye and as though it had taken a lifetime to get to this particular point in time.

The truth was that I couldn't wait to meet him. My desire to set eyes on a person whose feet had never touched the ground was overwhelming. Soon enough his introduction to the world would begin. His feet would touch the ground and, what's more, I would be the one holding him when it happened. Those little feet, maybe as brown and flat as mine, suspended over grass thinned by summer. It was time to admit not just my bottomless need for this baby but my desire to be a mother, so deep and unmentionable it was more like desperation. Once confessed, it could only grow. The future with a baby in it had long been written in my mind if only I could summon the bravery to look there. The images on cards I kept filed away, the memories of the future waiting to be taken out and played with like the toys of my own childhood. Kept, always, in the undisclosed hope that one day I might have cause to take them out again. I had obsessed over that scene in *All About My Mother* because it expressed that unspeakable need that had been in me since I was a child, not so long out of the womb and already tucking my teddies up in bed and whispering stories into the sucked fur of their ears at night. There was no reason or justification for it. I simply wanted to be a mother in the same unquestionable way that I wanted to live.

It was as though this baby had been produced, like the women remaking themselves in *All About My Mother*, by an act of will played out over years, a script written on my belly that I was only now learning to read. I had wanted this baby for so long. I had spent my life hoping him into existence, which was probably why now, when he was suspended on its brink, I couldn't bear to admit to it. But if I did, there it was, strong and palpable, the desire you harbour so long and companionably that you forget it is there at all. The heartbeat you don't notice until it speeds up. The breath you feel only when you hold it, then let go. It was the most famous line of *All About My Mother*, spoken by a transgender person, a woman who was born a man, performing alone on a stage: 'You are more authentic the more you resemble what you've dreamed of being.' I had always dreamed of being a mother.

Eight

June

We shall be monsters, cut off from all the world; but on that account we shall be more attached to one another.
Frankenstein, Mary Shelley

Egg-shaped, womanly sounding and named after the old Norse for wolf, the island of Ulva lies off the deeply scooped west coast of Mull in the Inner Hebrides. It is separated by the narrowest of straits, a channel so slender it seems more road than waterway. The kind one can imagine nipping across with a leap rather than a boat. Unsurprising then that Ulva's cattle were once swum over to get to the mainland market. The crossing over this sound is so short that one summons Donald, the boatman waiting on the opposite shore, by revealing a little red panel on a handwritten board. A necessary act in order to get from one place to another that is the most satisfying of island rituals. The board is located on a small stone pier at the end of a long ribbon of road beside Ulva primary school, its location on Mull rather than the island after which it is named demonstrating just how closely connected these two places are.

On a fiercely hot day in my eighth month of pregnancy I found myself standing on that baked pier, my lower back aching and my belly vaulting so triumphantly I could no longer tie my shoelaces without the most absurd of efforts.

Expecting

I pulled the panel across the slat until, with the tongue cluck of old wood, it flashed red. I watched as the little ferry anchored on the opposite shore perked up like a dog whose lead had been produced and began the two-minute journey over to pick us up. Us. Two women, one of them heavily pregnant, and an anxious Staffordshire bull terrier cross, tail curled between her legs like a jug handle. A family in waiting.

This was our last holiday before the birth, what is known in the commercialised language of pregnancy as a babymoon. A twenty-first-century mash-up of a word cannibalised from 'honeymoon', whose root refers to the period of sweetness experienced by newlyweds and, rather more cynically, the changing aspect of the moon. No sooner does it wax, in other words, than it begins to wane. As the travel guides, websites and top-ten lists would have it, a babymoon was a romantic and relaxing break for parents-to-be. A vision of rest and rectitude, whispered conversations about an unimaginable future in tautly made beds, last-minute love-making, floating belly-up in undisturbed pools, and always, always the onward march of afternoon teas. As far as I was concerned, a babymoon was closer to a visit to a place where I might lose myself and shake things up a bit. To its metaphorical meaning: a trip to the moon.

Perhaps it was because I was approaching full moon myself, a time in the lunar cycle when it is still claimed – no matter how strenuously scientists disprove it – that more babies are born. Conception, fertility and menstruation, which also shares a monthly cycle with the moon, have long been linked to its phases, the gravitational pull of this long anthropomorphised and poeticised satellite acting not just on the ocean's tides but on an individual's watery undercurrents too. What James Joyce refers to in *Ulysses* as the moon's 'potency over effluent and refluent waters: her power to enamour, to mortify, to invest with beauty, to render insane ...' And in the case of a pregnant woman, to break her waters. The moon tugging on the womb's high tide, causing the amniotic pool to burst its banks.

Midwives and doctors often speak anecdotally of labour wards being particularly busy on full moons and in one study of a hospital close to the tidal river of the Thames, the results revealed there were indeed more births when the moon was at its fattest. This theory, known as the lunar effect, would have held no sway prior to my pregnancy but now I found it mesmerising. There was something else, too. The dark side of the moon, its power 'to render insane'. The idea that its influence on a body (and a female body especially) that is four-fifths water could reach into her mind. Insanity had long been associated with the moon's monthly phases of exposure and concealment, light and shadow: 'lunacy' is derived from the Latin 'Luna'. Moon, woman and madness: a constellation shaped over centuries with pregnancy and birth as its brightest stars. And labour, in humans and animals, does tend to kick off during the night. Beneath an indifferent moon. Birth as the unsettling night-hour when women get down on all fours and bay at the moon, bright-eyed and instinctive as wolves. A time that, however inaccurately and harmfully, had long been associated with lunacy and used to pathologise, diagnose and incarcerate women.

The word 'hysterical' derives from the Latin *hystericus* meaning 'of the womb'. The nineteenth-century view was that insanity was passed down the female line and began, in other words, in utero. Women, habitually told nothing of what pregnancy and confinement actually entailed, were seen as morally weakened by the gravid state. Birth was characterised by some male doctors as a temporary period of insanity. And why wouldn't women be driven mad by an experience unknown, agonising and shame-laden, one that claimed so many lives and drove so many others to distraction? For the Victorians, parturition was the pinnacle of instability and a wide variety of responses to birth – from the malnourished mother of seven who hallucinated when she breastfed her newborn to the despair of the young woman forced to give up her illegitimate baby – were referred to under the catch-all umbrella of 'puerperal insanity'. And so it went on, the further back one travelled in human history. The belief in the 'wandering womb', taught by Hippocrates, continued for centuries; a condition in which the uterus was thought to float within the female body 'like an animal within an animal', causing everything from sleepiness to hysteria. The surgical removal of the uterus, still known as a hysterectomy, was routinely performed to treat 'female hysteria'. As though the womb was not only the origin of life, but of its unreason too.

All of this was abhorrent to the twenty-first-century woman landed on Ulva in her thirty-fourth week of pregnancy. Yet something was growing in me alongside the baby. A kind of unmooring was taking place, not from myself but from the world around me. I felt like a horse about to bolt. I had never experienced impatience like it and it expressed itself in an actual incapacity to stay put. Not just a need to get from one piece of land to another, but from one week to the next. I needed to fill time up so that it moved faster. I needed this nine months to be done. 'If pregnancy were a book,' Nora Ephron observed in her semi-autobiographical novel *Heartburn*, 'they would cut the last two chapters.' By the time I stepped on to Ulva, at that particular point in my own waxing phase, I was unravelling. My babymoon did become a kind of metaphorical journey to the moon. On my trip to the islands of Mull, Iona and Ulva, I went a little mad.

My pregnancy had been bookended by islands. Two of them, so different in character, climate and position, protruding from opposite hemispheres of the earth. They were like pillars rising out of two great oceans. South and north. East and west. One surrounding the country of my parents' birth, the other of my own and, in a few weeks, the next generation. The cultivated paradise of the Maldives in my first trimester, that secretive time when dry land swayed beneath my sea legs and the foetus swilled in my imagination like a tadpole in a jar. Now the expansive, robust and mountainous island of Mull in my last trimester, a time of slowness, bigness and excess.

The poem 'Islands' by Muriel Rukeyser, the Jewish American poet whom Anne Sexton once described as 'the mother of everyone', is a curt retort to all who have claimed that every man is an island. 'O for God's sake,' Rukeyser writes in the fabulously tetchy first line, 'they are connected underneath.' Although these two pieces of land were detached in almost every sense, if you opened your mind and let the world rush in they did indeed meet on the ocean floor. Now they seemed to heed Rukeyser's call and glimpse each other across the earth's own linea negra, the equator. It was as if my pregnancy had nudged them closer together, not just in my memory but on the map. They had been reconfigured in a few short months – less than a heartbeat in her ancient history – and from now on would always be connected by the causeway of my pregnancy. 'They look at each other / across the glittering sea / some keep a low profile,' writes Rukeyser. 'Some are cliffs / The Bathers think / islands are separate like them.'

Expecting

With three other couples, including my sister and her partner James, we stayed in a house on Mull that had been in the so-called 'current' family's ownership since 1865. It was just the right side of shabby, stuffed to the gunnels with old furniture, rugs, books, paintings, ornament and a family of swifts and housemartins knocking about in the rafters that woke me at the same dawn hour as the baby started kicking. I associated the house with the walk up three flights of stairs to get to our bedroom, which made my breath short and my heart knock against my chest. So much space in the house, the view across the Sound of Mull, the northern skies, and this volcanic hunk of land referred to by Ptolemy two thousand years ago as Maleos. Mull, perhaps from *meall*, meaning a lump, globe, rounded hill, mound or swelling. An island that had inspired Robert Louis Stevenson to write *Kidnapped* and Felix Mendelssohn to compose an overture. All this and yet so little room in this overstuffed house of mine, bustling with blood and activity.

The baby now weighed up to 5lb and was around 32cm from crown to rump and up to a staggering 45cm from head to toe. His sucking reflex was establishing itself and perhaps in secret knowledge of those little lips pursing in utero I began to wake up in the morning with a damp patch of milk – or colostrum as the first distillation of this lifestuff is known – on my T-shirt. It shocked me. Eight months in and I still wasn't ready for the bleeding obvious. One evening I got into bed and felt a long, slow clenching around my belly as though a belt was being tightened, hole by hole, across what I would once have called my midriff. A Braxton Hicks, the body rehearsing uterine contractions in the same way an opera singer marks a score without singing out. It did not hurt and the fact that I didn't have another one made me doubt, minutes later, whether it had happened at all.

The baby's coat of lanugo had almost shed itself (where did all that silken hair go? Did it dissolve back into the liquid dark of the womb?) to reveal what I imagined to be skin as soft and hotly perfumed as the underside of a puppy. The thick layer of vernix was, to my mind, like a warm and impressible coat of candle wax, encasing his body like a seal. His kidneys were done, his fingernails full length. In this final trimester, 250mg of calcium would be invested on his ever-hardening skeleton every single day. His lungs were almost mature – it would not be long before he could breathe independently of me. Before life outside the womb, with all its bright lights, jeopardies and polluted, oxygenated air, would usurp hibernation within. Before my body would beat with a single pulse again.

The baby was head down – I knew this both from the low-lying blip of his hiccups and my thirty-two-week scan. The vertex position, in which 95 per cent of babies are born. My ribs felt the difference the most, as if the tiny monkey feet prising them apart had got bored and the doors to the cage could creak closed again. The volume of my blood had reached a peak of five litres and hosting all that rich plasma was like standing on the bank of a rapidly rushing river. I felt acutely aware of the beat of my heart. Arrested by my own resting pulse.

I could breathe more normally, but the baby's descent had gravitational consequences. I began to experience the animal gnaw of pelvic girdle pain as he dropped and my body's scaffolding, beginning to soften with hormones, felt as though it might buckle under the load. The boat crammed with too much cargo. Still so far to go before anything could be jettisoned. The fatigue of carrying this much weight, of bailing and refilling my own body with this much blood, was on occasion engulfing. Twice in a fortnight I had a migraine, a terrifying headache unlike any other I had experienced. Haloes shimmered around my eyes like two tiny eclipses, blotting out wellness and light. Unnervingly pretty in their revolving hypnosis, they made me feel as though the only thing that could get in was hysteria.

The house was located on Mull's east coast in a tiny village called Aros, set way back from the road to Tobermory, Mull's capital, with its row of little painted houses overlooking the harbour in which yachts as white, sleek and well travelled as aeroplanes anchored in summer. A view so picturesque one struggled to look at it without the neat white frame of a postcard materialising around its edges. Like the superimposed experience of pregnancy, one had to go there to get beyond the frame.

Aros was most famous for its castle ruins on a blasted promontory that had been overseeing the noisy business of the river Aros meeting the Sound of Mull since the thirteenth century. The castle was a short walk from the house. So was the loop up to an Iron Age fort and on to a vast sea loch almost bisecting the island in two. So was the evening stroll down to the river to watch otters. I never saw any of it. This was to be a trip of unseen sights, unfinished walks and unrevealed nature. Where in previous months the world had assaulted me with its noise and stench, it now seemed to retreat like a wild animal. Entire landscapes stripped back to the fundamentals of road, water, hill and sky.

Claire and I drove about the island like retired pensioners and did short walks on forest trails or around lochs. Circular walks were abandoned before we reached the halfway mark, usually following the same conversation. Claire's sensitively couched suggestion that we should turn back, my stubborn and rather childish refusal, the silent attempt to forge on with tension and my belly heavy in the air, and then finally the admission. Yes, I was too tired. We should turn back. Defeat.

One morning we walked through Aros park from Tobermory with my sister and James, a moderately steep muddy track with views over to the Ardnamurchan peninsula where Claire and I had once spent a stunned week after my mother was diagnosed with breast cancer. I huffed and puffed at the rear, stopping to perch on logs and eat another dreaded biscuit or banana. The dryness of a mouth dehydrated by biscuit crumbs and the sweet-ripe squelch of a banana: two of the strongest body memories of pregnancy. I stood and watched James swim in the sea and felt like a mother. The one who keeps to the water's edge, never gets further than a paddle, stays beside the abandoned clothes, waits for the adventurers to return. The exercise of patience. Sitting out, watching more, participating less: perhaps it had begun already and pregnancy was merely a practice run for parenting. We wandered around a loch festooned with giant water lilies in a circle that never seemed to close. Eventually I admitted defeat and my sister and I waited in a car park, talking on a bench and watching the tits and chaffinches, while Claire and James went back for the car.

On a day trip to the island of Iona, a centre of pilgrimage for centuries with a piercing clarity of light and air, I insisted on taking the dog as we walked through a meadow sprayed with buttercups of such bright yellow that it seemed unfathomable that a colour like this had ever come to be associated with weakness or cowardice. The field descended to the coast, where it petered out to wild machair, dunes, a wide stretch of beach and finally sea. We spent a dreamy afternoon shell-seeking and paddling in the waves until the water slapped my belly and I felt guilty about the baby dunked without warning in the freezing sound of Iona. On the way back there were lambs in the field and Claire made to take the dog, who was already pointing an impatient paw, ears cocked, hungry for the chase. Despite all this, I insisted on keeping hold of her. Within moments she had yanked so hard on the end of her lead that I stumbled forward, ran a few comical steps, then went down. My reflexes kicked in and I dropped the lead, sank to my knees, and slammed my hands to the earth, my belly quivering in the dust. As Claire ran off in hot pursuit of the dog, who was running ever-increasing circles around the sheep, tears of shock and frustration came to my eyes. The meadow swam into a recriminatory haze of yellow. The colour of weakness, after all. What if I had fallen and gone into early labour on Iona? What if I had hurt the baby? It was a moment that, despite not actually happening, haunted the rest of my pregnancy. I would play it over and over again, reworking the ending like a masochistic director. The stumble, the staggering run, but this time the refusal to let go of the lead. The fall, hard and fast. The impact of my belly thumping down on warm earth. The bleat of the lambs. The buttercups nodding in the clearest of air. Then what? Contractions? Pain? The ceasing of movement in my womb? My mind would take me only so far.

There was so much that I could not do. Or rather everything I did do became lesser, harder and closer to home. Pregnancy distilling the world, making it smaller. The last months were like old age. A camaraderie with the end of life just as one was toiling on its beginning. The mind scaled mountains but the body sought sea level. I lumbered slowly, wisely, obliviously, in my own time. I was always judging the gradient of ascents and seeking out the nearest place to go to the toilet. I didn't entirely understand what was going on around me and didn't always care. I was usually slightly uncomfortable in my surroundings. I sat on a lot of benches as one does in the twilight of one's life.

Meanwhile the others stayed young. They went on uphill hikes to lighthouses, gorged on shellfish platters in Tobermory, stayed up late drinking whisky and wine, and took long boat trips to outlying islands. They returned with photos on their phones: a white-tailed sea eagle perched far away on a post, a colony of puffins encountered while belly-wriggling right up to the cliff edge. The puffins were one thing – I was to spend a week on the islands without seeing a single one of these ubiquitous chubby-cheeked comedians – but it was the belly-wriggling that really got me. It had been so long since I had lain on my stomach, chin cupped in hands, the length of me pressed to the ground. The thought of doing it was so subversive it made me wince even to imagine it.

Everyone who went to Mull went to Staffa, an uninhabited volcanic island rising in perfectly petrified hexagonal pillars of basalt formed from cooling lava sixty million years ago. From a distance or in photographs they looked like Venetian blinds carved from black rock, their texture as closely knitted as whale baleen. I do not know what they look like up close because I have not seen them, but it was in 1829 after encountering these geometric sculptures at Fingal's cave, a cathedral-like sea cave known for its ability to produce eerie shanties composed by wave and wind, that Felix Mendelssohn wrote home to his sister with the first notes for 'The Lonely Island', what later became his *Hebrides* overture. 'In order to make you understand how extraordinarily the Hebrides affected me,' he wrote, 'I send you the following, which came into my head there.'

Expecting

It was on the day our party visited Staffa that Claire and I went to our own lonely but rather more accessible island. Ulva, home to sixteen people, no roads or cars, a fine Thomas Telford church, basalt cliffs known as The Castles that are overshadowed by Staffa's more famed examples, and the kind of melancholy quiet that clings to any place that has long been abandoned. And Ulva has been left and sought for centuries. By 1840 the island was home to almost six hundred people and a thriving kelp and potato farming industry. Eight years later, the potato famines and clearances decimated the population to a hundred and fifty. Three-quarters were deported by the island's new owner, Mr Francis William Clark, in just four years. Families turned out of their cottages without warning, their thatched roofs set ablaze and their livestock scattered. The population has continued to dwindle ever since. The history scored on the landscape in its place names, like the settlement of Aird Glass where crofters were sent if they were too old, infirm or disabled to leave for the mainland or to sail to Canada and North America. This patch of boggy coastline strewn with winkles, seaweed and the ruins of their homes is still known as Starvation Point.

Life on the island dates back further still than the Vikings, who arrived in 800 and allegedly gave Ulva its name. There are megalithic standing stones that might have left the Vikings scratching their heads, and as recently as the 1980s archaeologists from Edinburgh University excavated remnants of a shell midden in a cave that indicate Ulva was inhabited from as early as 5650 BC. In this cave, named after the Scottish missionary David Livingstone, whose grandparents ran a small croft nearby, they found limpets, periwinkles, crab claws, flint artefacts and the charred fragments of bone from an Arctic fox, a lemming and a human infant. A neolithic stash described in the concise and resonant language of archaeology notes as 'pleistocene funeral remains and possible food processing area'. And if people lived, ate and died on Ulva seven thousand years ago, they were born on its terraced igneous rock too. Not just born, but birthed. A point that remained moot until you found yourself wandering the island with a belching boy in your own volcanic dome, and then the bare bones of that human infant grew flesh. What was its birth story? How did it end up in that cave? And what became of its mother, a woman with breasts, womb, cervix, perineum and birth canal not so different from my own?

Claire and I wandered off the boat at Ulva in a stupor, a punch-drunk state that seemed to characterise this eleventh-hour stage of pregnancy. We stupidly decided not to stop at the Boathouse for refreshments (in other words, I was too impatient to get going), found a path and took it. The ground was cracked, sandy and embedded with dusty stones. This, combined with the bleached white of the midday sun, made me feel as if we were on a Greek rather than a Hebridean island. There must have been a lot of rabbits running about in the reams of bracken because the dog pulled at the end of her lead, her eyes bulging and her tongue flapping like a sail. We did not dare let her off: she looked like she might never come back. We had no water and I kept fixating on her panting rather than on my own thirst. We had no map either, nor any idea where we were going. At first this didn't matter. The island was small, less than 5km wide at the amplest point of the oval. We walked slowly, cheerfully, saw no one.

It was not long before the red noise of my pregnancy began to disturb the peace. A need in me swelled ravenously until it obliterated everything else. I wanted to see the sea. To paddle in cool water. Though we had only just crossed over the sound, and I had only just trailed my fingers through its limpid waters, it did not count. I had yet to feel it close around my calves like a parent's comforting hand on your shoulder. I wanted to press my fat feet into sand, smell salt and seaweed, and hang over my own belly and beachcomb for shells. This desire was not sophisticated and knew nothing of history or wildlife. I did not yearn for a particular stretch of sand, coastline or view of The Castles. I had no interest in scanning the ocean for cetaceans or scouring the rocks for seal pups. It did not occur to me that I might see puffins after all. Or that I should keep my eyes peeled for the Slender Scotch Burnet moth with its paint splotches of red on a dandy's velvet jacket of jet-black wings. A creature that is no longer seen anywhere on earth but on Ulva and Mull during the months of June and July. I knew nothing of the island's history of private ownership and clearances, or the ruins of its sixteen abandoned villages. I had no idea that Johnson and Boswell, during their famous tour of Scotland's Western Isles, made the crossing to Ulva in 1773, calling for the boatman just as I had done, though 'the wind was so high that the people could not hear him call; and the night so dark that they could not see a signal. We should have been in a very bad situation,' Boswell continued, 'had there not fortunately been lying in the little sound of Ulva an Irish vessel [which] ferried us over.' I was like a child, stroppy and fatigued with nature for not producing her riches when I demanded them. Worse, I had the nimble impatience of a child coupled with the overstretched heart and bad temper of an old person.

Heading vaguely east we wandered around the small Telford church with its austere T-plan design, stacked school chairs, and dust motes falling in the fleshy light of its pale pink walls. We took photos of the latticed patterns drawn in shadows by the leaded windows and picked our way around the overgrown garden. I went through the motions, doing all the things that people do when they visit places that are not their own, feeling completely removed from my pre-pregnant self, your average guidebook bore who would have been reciting dates, descriptions and Johnson and Boswell quotes by this point. Instead I was quiet, at least on the outside.

Afterwards we ascended a rough track into a wood thickly carpeted with bluebells. The purplest of prose scrawled on the forest floor, known in Scotland as harebells and often an indicator that you are walking in ancient woodland. I had never seen so many of these droopy violet flowers with their little flouncy skirts in my life. And I had never been so unaffected. The blue of those bluebells, so blue it was as self-evident as the orange of an orange, was a mere backdrop to my own nature show.

For it was here that I lost it. Properly. I screamed and stamped and cursed and made a fabulously blue spectacle of myself. I stormed out of the dark woods onto the brow of a sunlit moorland and the light did nothing to dim my rage. I sat down heavily in the middle of the path, a protest of one with a cause unknown to myself. Yanking my balloon of a body to the ground sent the dog spare and she jumped all over me, tried to hump my back, licked my hands in front of my face, salty with tears rather than seawater. This of course made Claire laugh, and then I really bawled. For everything. I wept because I had blown my last chance to swim in wild water before the birth, howling as grandiosely as if I was mourning the time when all beings gave birth in the sea.

Expecting

I cried because I had never felt so massively fed up – nor so massive. I cried for my exhausted and invaded body, for the future I could not conceive, for the mother I might not become, for the child I would no longer be, for the baby I still could not claim. It was the most pleasant scene imaginable in which to have a hissy fit, the sun washing the moor into a spotlight for my performance. Eventually, after I had chewed all the scenery and spat it out, we headed back to The Boathouse, where I gorged on langoustines and oysters fresh off the boat in vengeful defiance. I was sick and tired of missing out. If I couldn't swim in the sea, I would at least snap up its fruits.

I had to accept it. I was heavily pregnant, my goose was nearly cooked, and I was mad. Deafened by the world within my body, so loud it was now blotting out the one beyond its skin-wall just as that migraine had eclipsed the light. A world that, for now, was thwarting me and had to be let go. It could not touch me with its tragedies and bluebell woods. It would have to wait. I felt cut off, set adrift, island-like and yet an anchoring had taken place. The umbilical cord was still tethered to my womb. The islands were connected at the ocean floor if you dived deep enough. '[A] plunge into the cold water of a mountain pool seems for a brief moment to disintegrate the self,' writes Nan Shepherd in the penultimate chapter of *The Living Mountain*. 'It is not to be borne: one is lost: stricken: annihilated. Then life pours back.'

The hysteria of your average pregnant woman was not the kind that needed to be diagnosed or used as a whip with which to beat her. It needed only to be felt. Hysteria not as a female condition but as a waxing, revealing phase of pregnancy. A necessary madness, as bare-faced, scarred and glamorous as a full moon. It was not hysteria in the historical and misogynistic 'female' sense, but it did belong to women because ours were the bodies that did the hard graft of forging life. Rather, it was a heightened insight in the same way that a palpitation is a hyper-awareness of the heart. A temporary immersion in time, body and self that was not an escape from reality but a slow walk towards it. To the island of the body that, once the baby had abandoned its fiefdom, would be left to itself again. It could not last, this madness, but while you were there you could go for it. Perhaps the hysteria of pregnancy was not madness at all. Perhaps it was merely the most appropriate and brave response to living and hosting life at its heaviest. 'All extremes of feeling,' wrote Virginia Woolf, 'are allied with madness.'

On the crossing back to Mull, life did pour back. Unbelievably, there was another heavily pregnant woman onboard the ferry. She sat with her partner, both of them looking straight ahead, her belly so full-mooned that the crater of her belly button had popped out. The boat was small enough that our knees were almost touching. Perhaps it was mere projection, like our propensity to see a face in the moon, but I felt a weight of emotion, expectation and hysteria on that boat. My eyes, red and hollowed out with crying, locked with hers and we shared an unsmiling look of comradeship, the way hikers nod at each other on a walk. I asked her one question: how far along are you? She was thirty-three weeks, just one behind me. We might have conceived at the same time, under the same moon.

By the time we were delivered to Mull a minute later I felt strangely calm. Perhaps it was the straightforward relief of having an unhinged episode on an island: one could leave it behind more easily. Perhaps it was the relief I always feel when I set foot back on the mainland, which is what the island of Mull felt like after our strange expedition. The city girl in me was always unable to resist the security of a wide, populated land mass. The simple reassurance that comes with a light from a stranger's house. A car on the road. Or perhaps it was the connection in seeing someone else stranded on an island of her own for nine months. The equivalent of waving to each other from our little protrusions of rock, not to shout for help but to say *I am here too.*

Later, much later, when the baby in my belly was a boy, my boy, throwing cushions to the floor and running fire engines up the arms of the sofa, I studied a map of Ulva. I traced the meandering curve of our route with my finger and saw that the point where it abruptly ended with my heavy seat on the path was not far from Livingstone's cave. A finger pressed to a dot on a map was enough to bring the memory of it all back in a flood of bluebells, white light, a red panel and a sea of salted tears. I thought of Ulva fondly, as though I could connect to that abandoned piece of land only once I had left it myself. I thought of that cave a few steps on from my sylvan meltdown. I thought of those tiny bones of fox, lemming and human infant. Of the bones not so chemically different from the rock of the cave that had held and protected them for so long. Of how they were loved, scorched and mourned by mothers and fathers seven thousand years ago.

Nine

July ... August

No gasp at a miracle that is truly miraculous because the magic
lies in the fact that you knew it was there for you all along.
Beloved, Toni Morrison

We drove down the east coast in silence, the most familiar
of drives so pregnant with portent that it took the words
from our mouths. One by one the everyday sights slipped by,
dipped in the yolk of a particularly beautiful sunset. The car
showrooms, business parks, industrial estates and dog and
cat home of unnoticed, unpeopled Seafield briefly gilded in
gold. The sea as still as a pond and coated, it seemed from my
vantage point whizzing by in the passenger seat, with a thin
film on which one could watch, upside down, the drama as it
unfolded in the sky. On the horizon I could just make out the
curve of the route we were driving with two out of three dis-
tinctive landmarks visible in the haze. The mighty Bass Rock,
home to the world's biggest northern colony of gannets for
much of the year, was for now excised but there, to the right,
was the perfect cone of the Berwick Law, once the spewing
open mouth of a volcano and now a moderate hill for climbing. Further along still, Cockenzie power station, with its tur-
bine hall and twin chimneys like cigarettes pulled from the
pack. Two perfectly symmetrical landmarks, one forged by
nature and the other by humankind, each emitting a certain

brutish dominance over the coastline. Geographically, at least, we could see exactly where we were heading.

It was approaching 9pm on a Sunday night. The hour of after-dinner relaxation, BBC period dramas, hanging up a wash, taking stock before the start of another week. Not for us. Ever since I had sailed past my 22 July due date and continued hour by hour, day by day, night by night, to be irrefutably and increasingly pregnant, we had been existing outside the ease of social norms. The days of the week were an irrelevance. The nights were for wandering, not sleeping. We counted in additions as though the clock had stopped and we were living on borrowed time. Forty plus seven, eight, nine, ten … the portions of time curiously empty, suspended and identical, until it occurred to me that the baby might not come in July at all. An August birth had not crossed my mind, yet here we were, chasing the sun down the coast on the first weekend of the eighth month of the year.

There had never been a sunset like it and Claire and I said as much to each other in small, tired voices as we passed through the Victorian seaside town of Portobello. Never had there been such soft honeyed light, a sea so smooth, a sky so quiescent. There was no wind, which even in high summer along this stretch of coast is noteworthy. The world seemed unbearably kind, hushed, almost motionless, as though it was holding its breath. It felt maternal, and being pulled to its bosom made a child of me. It did not occur to me that it was not the sunset that was special nor the light that returned me to my childhood. It was the moment in my life at which I came to it. That is, almost forty-two weeks pregnant, fuller than full-term, dazzled, depleted, vulnerable, up for the fight, on the brink of everything from induction to motherhood. So it *was* an extraordinary evening for the jittery couple driving past in a secondhand car just bought for the occasion of becoming a family. It really was a sunset like no other. It was my last before going into labour.

Dusk comes late to Scotland in summer. By the time we left the house for our drive down the coast the sun was beginning its descent and we watched in the wing mirrors of the car as it appeared to fatten and blush deeper with each passing mile. There was an overwhelming sense of time running out. We kept looking for a place to stop and watch it slip into the sea, just as it had done yesterday and would do so again tomorrow. But this was the one we needed to mark and it mattered in the ridiculous and heartfelt way in which things that have nothing whatsoever to do with you occasionally do. It was as if the fact that time had run out in my pregnancy had become conflated with this particular sunset. Perhaps we needed to witness it going down to put a stop to things. Or rather, to get them going.

Eventually, a car park suggested itself off a quiet stretch of road between the towns of Musselburgh and Prestonpans, in the shadow of Cockenzie power station. An in-between place, the sort at which you might stop if you were a local wanting to walk your dog or fish off the rocks of the small bay, or a driver from the power station depositing some of the 3,000 or so tons of ash and dust produced daily by the plant, forming a series of ash lagoons that stretch all the way back to Musselburgh. We parked up where the ash lorries stopped to dump their loads, got out and walked across a small square of grass to the old sea wall. Beyond it lay the ocean at low tide, calm and compliant. Inside my heap of belly the baby lay still and stubborn. Earlier in the day I had felt some tightenings across my belly but now they had stopped. A different kind of stillness, representing the storm that would never break.

Expecting

There is a certain quality of light produced by northern summer sunsets that gauzes the world, softening everything in its reach. That evening it made the view back to the city in which I was about to give birth, the hump of Arthur's Seat, Leith, the harbours of Newhaven and Granton, and the route we had only just driven, as inspiring as an eighteenth-century Scottish landscape painting. It was as though the hormones relaxing the bones of my pelvis to allow for the baby's passage into the world were also softening the city that would receive him. I felt uncharacteristically pliable too; more loving, compassionate and kind than I have ever known. The only other times in my life when I have come close to such softheartedness have been in the first stupefying weeks of falling in love. We took a photo of ourselves on Claire's phone, a selfie of our last night on earth as ourselves that neither of us has since seen or been able to track down. In my mind's eye it is soft focus, golden, with the sun behind us painting a halo around our heads and shadowing our faces. We look tired, older than our years, happy.

It was all so lovely that it took a while before we realised something else was happening, much closer, on clumps of rock exposed by the low tide. A single seal, stretched into the most seal-like of U-bends. Nose and tail curved skywards, belly squelched to the rock, as poised and sturdy as a ballerina en pointe. It may as well have had a striped ball on the end of its nose, so absurdly circus-like was the performance. It was far enough away that I had to focus and blink hard to see it. If there had not been two other people down on the beach watching with their phones held aloft, perhaps for their own proof, I would have doubted it had happened at all. My exhaustion bordered on hallucinatory, so that I didn't altogether trust my senses. We drove home in the dark, quiet and elated. Somehow I knew that it would be my last night on earth quite like it.

I have since been back to that car park and walked that stretch of coastline without a baby in my belly. It is nothing like I remembered, both more and less than my previous encounter. For a start, Cockenzie had just been blown up in a controlled explosion watched by thousands, its chimneys lopped off and its silhouette on the horizon reduced to a menacing box. The ash heaps are now reconfigured as a burgeoning nature reserve. The car park is no longer a spot known only to locals (it had probably never been). Just a year after I saw the seal curled into a croissant, our little bay became part of the John Muir Way, a 134-mile coastal path stretching from Dunbar in the east, where the great naturalist was born almost two hundred years earlier, to Helensburgh in the west, where he set sail for America. This meant all the explanations and interventions of a well-funded new route. Walkers' and cyclists' signs pointing west (2½ miles to Musselburgh) and east (⅔ mile to Prestonpans). Clear paths through gorse and rosehip that could, in sections, easily accommodate a buggy or wheelchair. Information panels with maps, local history and reproductions of old photos.

Our scrubby bay had a name. Known as Morrison's Haven, from as early as 1526 it had been a thriving harbour, exporting coal, salt and oysters across Europe. There were clues dropped along the bay if you knew to look for them. A concrete roundel that was once the base for the light at the harbour mouth. The grassy knoll a few feet from our little square of grass that would have been the harbour basin. On the beach itself, what looked like a strip of rocks leading to the water was in fact the remnants of a pier. And among the driftwood, razor shells and rocks slippery with algae lay a history written in flotsam and jetsam. Broken pieces of glass, opaque and rounded by the sea. Halves of oyster shells, frilly, pearlescent and drilled with clever little holes. A piece of ceramic shaped like a boat with the numbers 1854 stamped on it. And most of all, bricks, everywhere I looked, some the colour of rust, others of wet sand. The older ones had softened over decades into the shape of big bath sponges and the stamp of the kiln that bore them was all but rubbed out. The younger ones were still marked and out here in a place where it was so difficult to tell where the mark of the human hand ended and that of nature began, the text read like the sparest of concrete poetry. BURGH. NIDDRIE. PRESTONGRANGE. The letters somehow standing for more than themselves.

You could read the history and find out that by the middle of the eighteenth century, glass and pottery manufacturers were totally dependent on Morrison's Haven for exports. That right up to the late 1920s ships were calling in at the Haven to load up 600 tons of coal and bricks. That the harbour was filled in during the 1960s and Prestongrange brickworks, once home to twenty kilns, closed in 1975. Or you could just go and have a root around on the beach. Though I knew none of this on that Sunday evening in August when we pulled into a random car park to watch the sun go down, the history was there all the same. It left its marks on the landscape in the same way that my pregnancy and birth marked my body and, indeed, my life: silently, privately, with atmospheres rather than words. Landmarks and stretchmarks. Tracks and scars. My body as a location where history had happened. Really, though, it was the bricks. The fact that we fired them from clay and shale, stamped them with places we had named, used them to build houses and cities and power stations, to make our mark on the world and protect ourselves from its ravages with roofs and walls. But in the end some of the bricks wound up back where they started. On the beach, their past eroded by the rough hand of nature, almost indistinguishable from the stone and mud that bore them.

I had by this point had two membrane sweeps and was on the brink of a third. A simple procedure routinely offered to induce labour, it involves the midwife inserting a finger into your vagina and sweeping her finger firmly around the bottleneck of your womb. The action separates the membranes from the cervix, releasing prostaglandins that may (or indeed may not) help labour to begin. A sweep can be performed only if the cervix is already beginning to open, thin and shorten (the first is known as dilation, the second and third by the rather more lyrical effacement). In other words, the body must already be about to go into labour if a sweep is going to have any impact. For many, including me for most of my pregnancy, this made them seem pointless. Why do anything to speed up a natural process that is already happening? Months earlier, when I had heard pregnant women discussing sweeps in my antenatal yoga class (often bemoaning the pain of them), I had resolved not to bother. I was against induction unless either I or the baby was in genuine medical need of it. However, by the time I was ten days past my due date, perfectly healthy and frantic, Sarah offered me a sweep and my view did a complete volte-face. Clearly I had not understood the nature of desperation in late pregnancy. I jumped at the chance.

I lay on my back with my legs splayed open. I no longer cared about the extreme discomfort of the position. I had developed a cavalier attitude and 'bring it on' was the phrase that now characterised my state of mind. First Sarah measured me. At forty weeks my belly measured 40cm. Now at forty-one, it was 41cm. This minimal and perfectly reasonable growth horrified me. That the baby was still fattening seemed to suggest, in my skewed logic, that he would never come out. He would simply grow and grow. I had already been told by a number of people, most of whose opinions I had not solicited, that I was having an enormous boy. Sarah, as ever, reassured me. 'His head isn't getting any bigger,' she sensibly pointed out. 'And that's the hardest part to birth.'

Sarah took her time finding my cervix, apologising as she started digging around, saying that it was 'quite far back'. A flashback to my first scan in a room as dark and thrilling as a cinema. The words 'tilted uterus' and a tiny cartoon fried egg flickering on a screen. Then Sarah's face broke out into one of her lovely, quizzical smiles. She had found my cervix and pronounced it a centimetre dilated. I felt inordinately proud of this invisible achievement. My body, at least, was beginning to think about labour, even if I had yet to feel a contraction. Then something else made me gasp in shock. 'I can feel your baby's head,' Sarah said with her finger still inside me, for all I knew stroking it through the amniotic sac. I was stunned, though it was the most obvious of facts – *there is a baby right there between my legs* – and I had carried this information around for nine months. You would think it had ripened into a fact by now but it still blew me away. There he was, suspended between my legs. A few centimetres of my body now separated me from pregnancy and motherhood. From one person and two. He was so nearly in the world it seemed preposterous that he didn't simply plop into it. 'What's he like?' I asked, as though he was a man she had just met in a bar. 'His head feels lovely and smooth,' was her intriguing reply.

I was instructed to go home, relax, and look out for what is known in the dramatic business of birthing babies as 'a show'. That is, the passing of the mucus plug, a nine-month build-up of discharge and blood that seals the baby in the vacuum of the womb. And sure enough, that evening I felt crampy and my underpants were stained with an aged and rusty coin of blood. But then, nothing. More discouraging peace and quiet. Having spent all those months willing labour not to come, fearing it, seeing the peak in the distance and turning away, I was now summoning it. Running towards it. Bouncing on birthing balls, begging for the pain to begin.

Meanwhile, our flat goaded us with its perfectly set scene. The Moses basket in the bedroom, a cellular blanket folded neatly on the fitted sheet. The vests, sleepsuits, mittens and hats washed and folded away in the drawers. Breast pads to soak up the milk, and maternity pads for the blood. (I had only recently discovered from a woman at my antenatal class that I would bleed for up to six weeks after the birth as my womb emptied itself of nine months' worth of blood, mucus and tissue – known as lochia – in what sounded like the period to end all periods.) The hospital bag was packed in the event of a transfer, most of the contents of which were completely pointless (the rose facial spritz, in particular, seemed farcical). The labour playlist was compiled. The vitamin K injection for the baby was in the fridge next to the mustard, and two large canisters of gas and air stood in the sitting room – a pair of sentries watching us until they began to look more like part of the furniture than weird medical interventions in our home. In the spare room, what would one day be *his* room, a birthing pool I had rented from a website was waiting to be unrolled and filled. The fire department had come and tested its weight and we had tested it for leaks, or rather Claire had, running a long skinny hose to the bath tap, returning from B&Q with various attachments while I looked on, brainless and bewildered. The props were all in their rightful places. All that was missing was the script.

At first I felt calm, reasonable, myself. I had finished work at thirty-seven weeks and planned to read novels, take long baths, watch a few seasons of *Breaking Bad*, cook, walk, sleep. But I could not settle to anything, not even a book, and the days – those last precious weeks of rest and solitude, as everyone delighted in reminding me – slipped through my fingers. It was neither a quiet time inside my head nor on the street. Outside our flat the road was being dug up for the laying down of Edinburgh's tramline, a Sisyphean project that had gone on for years and had, in the process, uprooted 290 skeletons outside an old churchyard a few doors down from us. The skeletons, deep red in colour and preserved in wooden coffins, turned out to be five hundred years old. The tram project would never come to fruition in our belea-guered part of the city and though I did not know this at the time, the futility of the works got at me as if I did. The grind-ing noise, dust and anxiety-inducing juddering of our floors as the innards of the street were ripped out drove me to dis-traction. While the ground outside was opened up, my body remained agonisingly, incomprehensibly closed for business.

I had always known that I would have a long pregnancy. I had asked Sarah at the start to move my due date back two days. My menstrual cycle is long, which is often associated with a longer gestation. I was prepared, yet I had no idea what fourteen days of waiting for some unknown sensation to present itself would do to me psychologically. Towards the end, an entire night would pass with only a couple of hours of sleep in it. The rest was taken up with prowling around the flat like some nocturnal creature, eating bananas, bouncing on my birthing ball and, back in bed, heaving my giant mass from one side to the other in a painstaking attempt at tossing and turning. I watched films alone at night. My regression continued and they were always the sunny, sweet, tried-and-tested ones of my childhood. Waiting to birth a baby appeared to be turning me into one. 'In India,' writes Jhumpa Lahiri in *The Namesake*, as a woman labours in a foreign land, 'women go home to their parents to give birth ... retreating briefly to childhood when the baby arrives.' I thought of my grandmother returning to her mother's house in Bangalore to bring my mother into the world. I felt homesick and very British.

All of the old wives' tales about bringing on labour naturally were now attempted in earnest: hot curries, pineapple, raspberry leaf tea, sex, nipple stimulation, driving over cobbles, walking ... I sniffed clary sage – an essential oil that may (or, as ever, may not) bring on contractions – with the fervour of a clubber taking poppers. The sight of my lonesome and vast shadow rippling up and down the wall as I bounced on my birthing ball in the dead of night is one of my strongest memories of those strange days.

By day I was more or less sanguine and accepted that he simply wasn't ready to come out. By night I sought a more sinister explanation, one I could wield against myself. Was it me? My body? My age? My life? I felt infected with a guilt that had been handed down through centuries of shaming and blaming women and which I now seemed powerless to resist. Or was it the baby? Was there something wrong with him? Why wouldn't he come out? In my imagination he sprouted into a ten-month monster, dry as a husk, bigger by the day. Frankenstein's wretch, gigantic, grinning and wrinkled, refusing to abandon my womb. And what was I, then, but his horrified and horrifying creator.

Frankenstein. There is perhaps no novel that speaks to the fear surrounding pregnancy and birth more intensely than a novel written two hundred years ago by a nineteen-year-old girl who was, for much of its creation, pregnant herself. Mary Shelley astutely, intuitively, even unconsciously, understood the thrill and terror of summoning maternity into one's life.

So much death surrounds the creation of Frankenstein, which came to Shelley in a terrifying dream that she embellished over a single fevered year. She was as motherless as her creation, Victor, the hubristic 'pale student of unhallowed arts', and the 'hideous phantasm' he in turn creates. All three are, in fact, abandoned children. Shelley's own mother, the radical feminist Mary Wollstonecraft, died ten days after her birth from septicaemia. Wollstonecraft's entire life, wrote Virginia Woolf, was an experiment, a word that cannot help but evoke Victor's own attempts: 'Mary was going to have a child. She was going to write a book to be called *The Wrongs of Women*. She was going to reform education. She was going to come down to dinner the day after her child was born. She was going to employ a midwife and not a doctor at her confinement – but that experiment was her last.' It is the spectre of Wollstonecraft, the grief-stricken atmosphere left behind by her absence, that hangs heaviest over her daughter's novel.

Frankenstein, as Wendy Lesser points out in her 1992 introduction, is, like *King Lear*, a world without mothers. Victor's mother dies soon after he goes to university and the monster, crucially, is motherless. Nevertheless, after a 'painful labour' that culminates, one dreary night in November, in 'an anxiety that almost amounted to agony', Frankenstein births his creature and almost immediately after abandoning him in 'horror and disgust', has a terrifying dream in which he cradles the corpse of his own mother. 'A shroud enveloped her form,' he recalls, 'and I saw the grave-worms crawling in the folds of the flannel.'

By the time Shelley sat down to write the book in Geneva during the summer of 1816 she was not just a daughter without a mother but a mother who had lost a child. She had already had two children with her lover, Percy Shelley. One, a girl, died a few weeks after the birth. The second, a boy named William (the same name she gives to the child who is murdered in the novel), died a year after the book's publication. And during the writing of her novel, Shelley was pregnant with a third baby, a girl called Clara. She died three months before Frankenstein came out.

Tragedy haunted the novel's gestation. Shelley began writing in June and in October her beloved half-sister Fanny Imlay committed suicide. The following month, Percy Shelley's wife Harriet killed herself. In the five years around the writing of Frankenstein, Shelley birthed four babies and lost three of them. 'Dream that my little baby came to life again,' she wrote in a journal entry in 1815, 'that it had only been cold, and that we rubbed it before the fire, and it lives.' A year later she was writing about a scientist who hopes to 'infuse a spark of being into the lifeless thing that lay at my feet.' It's an extraordinary amount of death, even for the time, and what's even more extraordinary, perhaps, is that out of it came the archetypal creation myth. The modern Prometheus. The story not just of a birth but of *the* birth; of science fiction, monsters, feminist consciousness and an age of industry and intellectual hubris that is now so woven into the fabric of our culture that the creator and his creature go by the same name. No wonder Frankenstein came to me in those skin-crawling days when I feared not just birthing a big unloveable monster but, perhaps, becoming one myself.

Friday. Two days after my first membrane sweep I had another one and there was progress of a sort. I was now 2cm dilated. So early labour was happening; it was just that I couldn't feel it. Sarah told me that if the baby had not come by Monday our home birth would be in jeopardy and I would need to consider induction. A hospital appointment was booked for Monday morning – though 'I'm sure the baby will be here by then,' she added – where I would be monitored and scanned to check the baby, the quantity of amniotic fluid and the health of my placenta, which at this stage could deteriorate fast. An organ dying in order for life to start. Saturday came and went and on Sunday we went to the Scottish National Gallery of Modern Art, the stolid neoclassical façade from which blazes Martin Creed's neon sculpture *Work No. 975: EVERYTHING IS GOING TO BE ALRIGHT* in electric blue.

There was a free exhibition on called 'From Death to Death and Other Small Tales' and we wandered around it halfheartedly. Only the last piece, by a Brazilian artist called Ernesto Neto, caught my attention. It was called *It happens when the body is anatomy of time*, reminding me of Muriel Rukeyser's description, in her series of *Nine Poems for the Unborn Child*, of the gravid body as 'a house that time makes'. I was, in that instant, as literal an embodiment of the anatomy of time as a clock on legs. Neto's piece was a big work, taking over an entire room of the gallery. Great columns in Lycra tulle stretched to fat pod-like feet on the gallery floor stained orange and red by spices encased in them. Clove, cumin and turmeric. The precise smell, warm and throat-catching, of my father's brown faux-leather suitcases when he returned from India. The bitterness of turmeric, a scent that stained my childhood as it coloured my mother's food, our fingers when we ate, and the vessel of boiling water we were given to breathe when we had a cold, into which a teaspoon of this bright orange spice was ceremonially stirred. It choked my throat like a memory. In that room was the smell of home, my parents and the motherland I had never really known.

Back outside, I wandered the permanent lawn sculpture designed by the architect Charles Jencks. Entitled *Landform Ueda*, the serpentine mound coils in an 'S' around a series of crescent pools and is usually home to children tumbling down the slopes, art lovers and tourists strolling the terraces and photographing the reflections of the gallery in the water. It is one of my favourite places in Edinburgh. 'If you look at the way nature organises itself, it has inherent principles of movement,' Jencks has said of *Landform Ueda*. 'I wanted to design something which reflected these natural forces but heightened them.' The hillocks, seen from the road, look a bit like burial mounds, but they could just as easily be gravid bellies. Another biological design that reflects natural forces but heightens them. Claire's sister, who had come with us that afternoon, laid her hand on my belly as we paused atop one of these turfed mounds and said she could feel my womb tightening and then releasing. A contraction. She took my hand, laid it there, and sure enough I felt it too. A clench, small and determined as a jaw. I watched more closely and waited, statue-still atop Jencks's sculpture. There it was, the lightest tremor, a hardening that manifested as a very slight pointing of the dome from classical to gothic, the kind that perhaps can be seen only if it is simultaneously felt. I had never expected to be able to *see* a contraction.

Expecting

That was the evening we drove down the coast. A last gasp of a day stuffed with life that ended with another sleepless night. This time it felt different. I stayed in bed, sleeping fitfully and rocking on my hands and knees when the mood took me. In the morning, exhausted but miraculously energised, we returned to the Hermitage, the old gorge where we had walked on the day I found out I was pregnant. Another season, another life. Despite my exhaustion I stomped the high paths as if I was an over-enthused fitness trainer leading an early-morning hike. A few times I had to stop, press my hands against the creased elephant-hide bark of a tree and groan. Were these contractions? If so, they were short, random and exciting. They didn't hurt but one came as such a surprise I dropped my brand new smartphone on the rough stony path. It landed softly on its face but when I picked it up and turned it over the glass was smashed to pieces.

11.30am. The Royal Infirmary for my check-up. In the busy but oddly quiet waiting area my contractions started for real. Short and punchy, just a few seconds long, with an accompanying ache humming across my lower back and sending little forks of lightning down my legs. We used Claire's watch to time them. Eight minutes. Ten minutes. Six minutes. Ten minutes. Every now and then I left the building and walked up and down the concrete circular space outside while the people in the waiting room watched my performance through the glass with mild interest. It seemed absurd that we were here to check on my progress when I was clearly in labour. *Look*, I wanted to scream in frustration and pride. *It is happening*.

Eventually I was seen. I was hooked up to a machine for an hour to monitor my contractions electronically. The same machine that would be used throughout much of my labour if I was induced. A tight band stretched around my belly pressing two transducers to it as a glass is held to a wall to spy on what's happening next door. One to monitor the baby's heartbeat, the other to track my contractions. These fat black discs were wired to a machine that blurted out information on a never-ending scroll of thin paper that reminded me of the smooth yet scratchy toilet rolls at my primary school. An unfathomable tale spewed out in peaks and troughs that appeared to be translating the action of my body into a language I didn't speak. In any case it confirmed what I already knew. I was in early labour. My contractions were roughly eight minutes apart. The baby's heartbeat was normal – between 110 and 160 beats per minute – and galloping faster with each contraction as though he, too, was running the marathon alongside me. This moved me to tears. I felt, perhaps for the first time, that we were in this together. From now until the end.

Next we saw a radiographer, a woman about whom I remember nothing except that she had a thick cloud of hair that reassured me inexplicably. She scanned my uterus – the last of five increasingly blurry scans throughout my pregnancy – and confirmed my placenta and the levels of amniotic fluid were healthy. I don't recall the images. I may not even have looked at the screen. At this stage, just one day before I would see this baby in front of my own eyes, watching him on a screen had entirely lost its power. Finally another internal examination. I was pronounced fully effaced and 3cm dilated.

I was booked onto the labour ward for an induction the following morning, by which time I would be fifteen days overdue. 'There is no way you will need it,' the midwife told me. 'I would put money on you going into active labour tonight.' The stakes were getting higher by the hour. That night would be my last shot at a home birth. She offered to do one last sweep and I agreed. By the time Claire and I had returned to the car park it had done its work: my contractions were coming on stronger, and I could feel the show soaking my underpants. The journey home was spent on the back seat, groaning on my hands and knees. There is a particular street a few miles from our flat that I can no longer drive up without feeling, viscerally, that I am in those triumphant early hours of labour once again.

4pm. Home. Claire's sister came to take away the dog, who was getting angsty. My contractions were about four minutes apart, so I asked Claire to phone the midwife, though neither of us was sure whether it was too soon. I went around the flat, closing our old wooden shutters one by one, feeling as if I was blowing out the candles in church. I put on yet another film from my childhood, Danny Kaye's *The Court Jester*, and don't recall watching it beyond the chirpy opening credits. The midwife came, not Sarah as she wasn't on call that night, but a Glaswegian woman called Gillian who had three boys of her own, all birthed naturally, a no-nonsense manner, laughing eyes and a few moles on her face that I would fixate on during the biggest of my contractions. She had just moved through from Glasgow and I was to be her first Edinburgh home birth. I had never met Gillian before but, like a puppy, I trusted her instantly and completely and followed her everywhere. She examined me – my first (and last) internal on my own bed – and pronounced me 4cm dilated. I was in active labour. Only a handful of sentences remain intact from the night that followed and this is one of them. *I'm going to be here with you now until you have your baby.*

Claire seemed constantly, admirably busy. She set up my TENS machine – rented from the Pregnancy and Parents Centre for a fiver – and strapped it to my back, turning the current up full so that I yelled at the shock. We laughed at the absurdity of a situation in which Claire was giving me electric shocks, and I was asking for them. There was still room to laugh. Still, the distraction that little box provided, from the actual buzzing of each shock to the constant fiddling with the dials, was better than any breathing exercise, aromatherapy oil or Duncan Chisholm song. It took my mind off two areas of deep gnawing pain: in my lower back and, less expectedly, in my thighs. I remembered something I had read in Ina May Gaskin's *Guide to Childbirth* – a book that had thrilled and frightened me in equal measure in those rather prudish early months of pregnancy. It was about a labour during which a group of midwives rhythmically pounded the women's thighs. It had struck me as a bit of a hippyish Seventies ritual but now I understood it perfectly. The need to be worked on by expert hands. To have strong-armed, been-there-before women knead your flesh like dough.

At some point the TENS machine was abandoned, as useless as a TV remote control. The birthing pool was filled and the lights were dimmed to a red glow. All of life telescoped into our sitting room with its sloping floors, collection of vintage tobacco tins and stacks of books. The hours began to pass unmarked. At some point we must have entered nighttime. There was, I noticed vaguely, music playing. Duncan Chisholm on repeat on our CD player, just as I had imagined. But it sounded as if it was playing underwater, at a party that was happening nearby but that had nothing to do with me. So where was I? Somewhere that looked like my life but knew none of its past. A wordless place, Lynchian in tone and mood.

Expecting

I begged Gillian not to leave me, not even to go to the toilet. I begged her for food (she later told me she had never seen a woman in labour talk about eating so much). I begged her for gas and air, that colourless, odourless mixture of oxygen and nitrous oxide also known as laughing gas. She kept refusing me on the grounds that the longer I waited the more effect it would have until eventually she agreed. She showed me how to suck on the mouthpiece attached to a handheld filter that, as soon as it was in my hands, I refused to give up. Nothing and no one could have prised that piece of kit from my fingers. I took it everywhere with me. When I had to leave it momentarily to go to the toilet, my contractions become enormous in both size and length. As soon as I sat on the toilet seat, a giant surge ripped through my uterus in anticipation of my bladder opening. The birthing pool had the same effect, the warm water making my contractions sprout like lilies. At the beginning of each one – and they were every couple of minutes now, each one lasting up to a minute – I put the mouthpiece between my lips like a bit and, white-eyed and indignant as a bucking horse, attempted to breathe as deeply and slowly as I could through to the end. It gave me something to do, somewhere to direct my breath and a container in which to deposit my rhapsodic growls. There were a few numbers and letters separated by a dash or two around the rim of the mouthpiece. This trivial stamp of officialdom became the secret code of my labour. 'Find something to focus on,' Gillian instructed, watching me from our sofa with her hands clasped on her lap and an expression of amusement masking concern that made her look like a mother watching her child in a school play. And seeing as I did everything she told me with absolute

168

obedience, I focused on the nearest thing to hand. The code right in front of my face. I read that jumble of numbers and letters more than a hundred times, probably to the point of appearing cross-eyed, as though my life depended on memorising its meaningless contents.

Those contractions felt at once shocking in their force and entirely familiar. I had never experienced them before yet my body knew them as intimately as a bowel movement, orgasm or drop into deep sleep. Like quickening, they felt exactly as they ought to feel. Each contraction, or surge, or wave or pang or whatever inadequate name we choose to give to the rhythmic tightening and shortening of the uterine muscles in labour was all-consuming in its power. An earthquake striking the globe with a black pitiless force, threatening to crack it open. Pain seems as useless a word to describe the ascent to the crest of each of these grave and majestic swells as love is to describe the network of feelings we have for the people in our lives. Black was its colour and the ocean its crowning metaphor: rhythmic, glittering, awesome and utterly indifferent to the woman watching open-mouthed and blown away from the shore. Perhaps this is why we want to birth in water, an element in which we can neither live nor breathe. There is something about its brute force that is perfectly suited to the smash and grab of birth.

At the other end of the spectrum, I felt like a machine. Hard, cold, manmade, designed to crush and compress in the same way cars are flattened to slabs in a junkyard. Later, a train at full speed: sleek and thunderous, impossible to stop. I was not in the driver's seat and I did not remotely care. 'Boarded the train there's no getting off,' wrote Plath in the breathless final line of 'Metaphors'. I felt dangerous. Labour made a different person of me:

smaller, braver, reckless as James Bond. I had never seen this woman before but I loved her. She had no past, future, and indeed by the following morning she would be gone, seamlessly replaced by yet another stranger. A mother. But this labouring woman was the most alluring. She knew no fear. She operated on pure instinct. She was constructed from roaring sensation, presence and sound. She was a warrior. For weeks after the birth I remained obsessed with her but she never did return.

The satisfaction and relief of letting go, expelling everything with neither shame nor awareness. Thought, sound, vision, intellect, personality, past, future: all were dumped like clothes on the beach before the mad dash into the sea. The release was rapturous and unexpurgated. The sweet childish warmth of releasing my bladder in the birthing pool. My growls, low, strange and guttural, making my throat sore between contractions as it used to get after a heavy night out. The quick and efficient vomit into a bowl that Claire held out for me. The surprise of realising that I was kneading Gillian's buttocks while I clung to her like a monkey. There was no fear, embarrassment or sense of consequence. That the point of all this was to birth a baby was entirely lost on me. There was only this and there would only ever be this. It was a complete tunnelling of vision and a magnifying glass on life that, for some reason, we have come to associate more with death than life. I was not the light at the end of the tunnel but the tunnel itself, a vacuum capable of pulling in and pushing out all life. 'The black force,' Plath had called it in her short but beautifully detailed journal entry on the birth of her son at home.

'Conserve your energy,' Gillian demanded. 'Control your pain.' I stared at her wordlessly. Felt immeasurably proud when she said, 'You're doing so brilliantly. You've no idea how well you're doing.' Claire's presence was reassuring, quiet, but somehow distant. If she went out of the room I demanded her immediate return. When she was there I ignored her. I cared for no one apart from Gillian, a woman who had entered my life only a few hours earlier but whom I had come to rely on more than anyone else in the world.

Now she wanted to examine me again. I refused. Lying on my back with her fingers seeking my cervix brought on huge contractions. She insisted and told me, speaking slowly and sternly as though I were a child (which, as far as I was concerned, I was), that I was getting tired and had been labouring for hours. If I had not progressed to more than 6cm dilated we should consider transferring to the hospital. She mentioned pain relief. An epidural. Words that suddenly held no fear. I was unable to respond but nodded. I felt defeated, alone and ready for the decisions to be wrested from my hands.

It was the most extraordinary moment of my labour. I lay on our rug, squirming and snarling like an animal that had just been captured. Gillian examined me swiftly between two almighty contractions and looked amazed. 'You're nine centimetres dilated,' she said. 'I think your baby is going to be here by midnight.' Their faces, looking down on me and then at each other. Pure exultation. Nothing more or less than the three of us in that room. Then, as if in celebration of this remarkable new piece of information, I had my biggest contraction yet. I sprang up so high it was as though I had been shot from a cannon towards the ceiling. And then my waters broke. A great flood soaking the rug, the pillows, my legs, everything. In my imagination it sloshed all the way to the walls, seeped into the cracks between the uneven floorboards.

Expecting

What then? The bullet train speeding up. The machine at maximum capacity. 'How much more of this?' I rasped from the pool. 'They're not long enough,' Gillian barked. 'They need to be ninety seconds at least by now.' The summoning of everything in my being. It worked. My next contraction, Gillian told me at the end of it, was ninety seconds long. After these monster surges subsided and the water in the birthing pool stopped thrashing, peace descended as eerie and unsettled as the ocean floor, and I felt exhausted and furious. There was my enormous belly still protruding from me, unchanged in shape or size. So much work and yet still it rose up, as massive and immoveable as a boulder on the flank of a mountain. 'The sight,' wrote Plath in her account of Nicholas's birth, 'glimpsed between lids opened for a split second, of my still frighteningly huge stomach which did not seem to have altered during all the hours.'

Then my heart rate increased in the birthing pool. Gillian used a handheld Doppler against my belly and discovered that the baby's had also gone up in tandem with my own – it seemed we did everything together – and ordered me to get out. It felt like a turning point. The beginning of things not going my way. Back on the rug, surrounded by a detritus of sheets and soggy pillows and draped over my birthing ball like a rag doll, I wept. 'How much longer?' I kept wailing. And then, for the first time, 'I can't.' 'Transition!' Gillian announced jubilantly, referring to the stage in labour when the body changes its focus from opening the cervix to preparing to push. 'You can. You are.' Claire joined in and they praised and patted me like a creature. I stood up on foals' legs. Beside our sofa, using the arm as leverage, I started to squat low and deep, wrenching myself back up again and ranting and raving. 'Come on,' I recall screaming. 'Get this fucking thing out of me.' Gillian told me that if I wanted to I could push. Another midwife now seemed to be in our flat. She wore glasses and had hands cool and smooth as glass. I heard Gillian tell Claire to go and get the Moses basket and baby clothes ready. I had no idea what was going on, no clue what pushing meant. Still the contraction-producing machine that had colonised my body grinded on. Started to bear down.

A while later, after squatting, returning to the pool, then coming out and pushing, sodden and enraged, on my hands and knees on the rug, Gillian examined me again, this time while I was standing. I did not see her face but I knew something was wrong. She disappeared and I heard her on the phone. She returned and told me the news. Devastation. The baby's head was stuck in some kind of sideways position. It was pushing against my cervix, thickening it up again. The black force of my labour, it seemed, was tunnelling back on itself. Sucking the world up. A puckered mouth rather than a gaping hole. Resistance. We needed to go to hospital and an ambulance was on its way. Gillian told me not to push, that I could damage myself, but it was an instruction as preposterous as telling a person not to breathe. I thought nothing, said nothing beyond a few expletives, felt only outrage. Couldn't stop pushing. Claire seemed very faraway, lost in other rooms or perhaps worlds, packing bags and sending text messages. Gillian, too, was busy gathering things. I felt abandoned. The second midwife, whose face and name I would never know, helped me into a pair of black leggings. I rested my hands on her shoulders, slowly stepped first one leg and then the other into soft black Lycra between contractions, reduced completely and willingly to a child dressed by her mother.

Within minutes the paramedics had arrived. A man and a woman who wanted me to walk down our two flights of vertiginously steep stairs. They could not carry me. It was too dangerous while I was in the height of labour. Those two flights of stairs, that I had run up and down every day for years, up which shopping, furniture and Christmas trees had been lugged, rubbish taken down, and buggies worried about incessantly throughout my pregnancy, now became the Everest of my labour. I have never felt so appalled at the prospect of doing something. No fear, just a fury almost as black and consuming as my contractions. Gillian waited at the bottom, Claire behind me. The paramedics attempted to hurry me along, for which (inside my head) I called them every name under the sun. Each step brought on an enormous contraction. Stop. A howl of rage into my gas and air. Another step. And so it went on until Gillian appeared around the corner, cheering me on as though she was behind a finishing line and I was charging towards it at full pelt.

Inside the ambulance I was strapped to a gurney lying on my side, foetal and furious. 'Stop pushing,' Gillian demanded. 'I can't,' I shouted. Now that I was working against my contractions, trying to slam the brakes on the train, turn off the machine, I was lost. Panic descended. Pain. The body swimming against its own tide. The same thing happened to Plath during Nicholas's birth. The midwife went from praising her pushing to telling her to stop because the baby had not descended far enough. 'The minute I stopped pushing, the pains made themselves felt, awful, utterly twisting.' From manageable to inconceivable, it changed as soon as I was told the baby was stuck. How could it be that the relentless cycle of contractions seizing and crushing my body was unproductive? There seemed, suddenly, to be no reason for them at all and this made them horrifying. I kept screaming that the baby was coming nonetheless, imagining his little wet head pushing up against my leggings. The first wail muffled by a mouthful of bobbly Lycra. Now and then Gillian put her hands inside my leggings to check. No baby. No head. Nothing. It didn't even seem as though he was in my body any more. There was only the machine, crunching on forever. Claire sat beside me, politely answering inane questions from the paramedics. I squeezed her hand as hard as I could, reaching out in fury as much as in support. I did not once let go during the rush to the Royal Infirmary, lights flashing and sirens blaring. A journey of miles, right across the city, north to south, that was over in a few minutes. I recall thinking, with a stab of excitement and horror, *I have never been in an ambulance before.*

1.30am. Inside the labour ward I kicked and screamed and swore and demanded an epidural. From home birth to Hollywood in one fell swoop. More amniotic fluid burst out of me when I was deposited on the bed and this time it was flecked with meconium. The baby's first faeces, dark green and algae-like. A sign that he was in distress, though I have also heard it is not uncommon for overdue babies to be born with some meconium in their waters. Everyone shouted at me to calm down. I felt hands all over my body. The drama felt almost choreographed in its extravagance, like some overblown and tasteless piece of site-specific contemporary dance. I yowled on like a wildcat. A doctor arrived. There was also a young, sweet-faced midwife who was very sympathetic to my frenzy and let me pummel her. Then Gillian dropped a bombshell. She told me that she would have to leave. Her shift had long finished and she was handing over to the doctors and midwives at the hospital. She was going home. I was appalled. 'Don't leave,' I whimpered, as though she was a lover about to walk out on me for good. 'I have to,' she said. And then I hardened, grew defiant, got sick of all the begging, adoration and abasement that had characterised our night together. 'Well fuck off then,' I hissed in her face. And that was it. She left without another word.

I was instructed to sit on the edge of the bed and stay completely still. Between contractions, which by now were virtually constant, I locked eyes with Claire, unblinking and savage, while an epidural was plunged into my lower back. I felt nothing. Emotionally, however, I was soon euphoric. The prospect of the contractions being cut short was nothing short of miraculous. There was no disappointment, fear or distress. Only delight as the drugs went to work and slowly, sublimely, I began to feel nothing from the waist down. The black force dulled. The machine turned not off but down to an imperceptible level. The sheer relief and joy of becoming myself again. I apologised to everyone in the room for arriving in such an unhinged state. I used words. Made sentences and jokes out of them. I turned to Claire and saw her, properly, for the first time all night. She looked dreadful. 'Are you all right, darling?' I asked. She burst into tears and threw up into my sick bowl.

The work felt done. I felt elated as though I held the baby in my arms, though he still 'mountained huge ahead of me', as Plath put it in her journal entry. I lay on the bed, monumental and passive as a beached whale, while a procession of doctors and midwives shook my hand then looked between my legs. I felt like a giant MacGuffin, filled with something bright and precious that I, mere audience rather than participant, would never be permitted to see. All I got were the expressions on their faces as they peered inside the cavern of my womb.

An electrode with a tiny wire was inserted into my cervix and placed onto the baby's head to monitor his heart. I felt so sorry for him. His soft new scalp, pricked and prodded. After a while his heart rate returned to normal, though it kept increasing whenever the cocktail of drugs being passed through a drip into my body was topped up. I hated them too, they made me shake uncontrollably. The drugs were reduced. He calmed down. The shaking abated. I was left then checked, left then checked. I kept telling everyone I still wanted to have as natural a birth as possible. Now that I could talk again it seemed I couldn't stop marvelling at the sound of my own voice. We signed forms about C-sections, epidurals, forceps and episiotomies. Got into an argument with the registrar about the latter. I refused to be cut, should the situation present itself. In a grim way, I was enjoying myself. I felt ready for anything. All the options were on the table. Choice, of the most limited and unwanted sort but choice nonetheless, had returned to my life. I was out of the black tunnel into which I had been falling, recklessly and repeatedly, for hours and back in the people-made world of forms, disagreements, options.

Finally, for the second time that night, I was pronounced fully dilated. And so, lying on my back with my legs open, I leaned forward and pushed as hard as I could. The midwife, consultant and Claire cheered me on. Told me I was a brilliant pusher. I became a warrior again, red-eyed and resolute. There was nothing, literally nothing, I wouldn't do to get this baby out of my body. I pushed until I thought my eyes would pop out of my skull. I felt nothing but a blissed-out doggedness and great pride at being the centre of attention. The consultant kept putting her hand inside me to check. I pushed again. The baby would not descend. I pushed again, angry with him now. My contractions were so strong, my pushing so A-grade. Still, he refused to budge. He was well and truly stuck.

Theatre. A room so white and dazzling it looked like the end of life. 'I've never been in theatre before,' I heard myself gasp. 'It's beautiful.' I felt calm and magnanimous and the fact that I was pumped full of drugs did not for a moment occur to me. I was profoundly moved by the sight of an anaesthetist, registrar, consultant, nurses and Claire, small and pale as a ghost in her scrubs, gathered here for me. A random group, all of whom had been born and some of whom may have given birth, who happened to be here on this night, at this particular hour of need for me and my baby. For suddenly that was simply and irrefutably what he was. Mine.

One by one they introduced themselves to me, an NHS formality that made me weep tears of gratitude. I told them how wonderful they all were. Praised the fortitude of the National Health Service. Implored them to take good care of us. Gazed up at the brilliant white of the ceiling and talked and talked in a monologue that felt scripted it was so seamless and long. Claire wept beside me silently, holding my hand as though she were the child and I the mother.

First, I was numbed all over again. I breathed in and began to count as puffs of cold air were sent down my body from top to bottom and a question repeated over and over again. Can you feel this? And this? This? Just below my chest the answer quickly became no. A little white curtain was erected halfway down my body. The anaesthetic made me retch repeatedly. The anaesthetist stroked my hair and called me darling. The tears rolled in a deluge from the corners of my eyes onto the bed. I was neither sad nor scared, just unspeakably moved.

I had insisted on a C-section as a last resort and so the consultant tried forceps first. The baby was still relatively high up in my pelvis so they were rotational forceps, giant salad servers out of a joke shop inserted deep inside me and turned this way and that to manipulate the baby's head into a better position. The consultant tugged me down the bed. It worked. The baby's head turned. But still, even with forceps, he would not be pulled out any more than he would be pushed. There was no path left to the top of the mountain, all ways obscured by the pristine whiteout, and now, for the first time, there was real danger. Urgency. The baby was in distress. The swift response of a medical team who know what they're doing but no longer have the time to share it with you. It was a C-section, and now.

I was sliced open expertly, routinely, felt nothing. The world seemed reduced to a series of small, astonishing facts in the way a single word, when placed alone on a line, becomes poetry. I was told not to worry if he didn't cry when he was pulled out because he might have too much fluid in his lungs. But then, in spite of this warning, came a cry, bold and loud, not belonging to this disinfected and orderly place but belonging so absolutely to him. 'A big healthy boy,' some-one pronounced. 'Lots of hair.' It was 7.02am on 6 August. Claire sobbed. I felt more deliciously, orgiastically exhausted than I have ever done in my life.

The baby was shown to us quickly but I was still heaving into my bowl and barely saw him. Oily black hair slicked to a head. Big white hands around a robust pink baby body. Little chicken legs pulled up. He was whisked away to have his lungs cleared. Perhaps this should have worried me, but I was so tired and relieved that he was out of me I lay there in a kind of glittering ecstasy. The doctor told me he would have to stitch me up as I had a small tear from the forceps. It was only then that I wept tears of devastation for myself, that my labour had ended like this, that I was a body that required stitching back together. I felt very alone for a while as Claire retreated to the back of the room to vomit into another sick bowl and, though I did not know it, hold our baby boy. I lay there, drifting in and out of sleep or perhaps consciousness, veering from relief to shock to awe at what I had just done. I had tried everything. I had seen myself in a way I had never done before. I felt very brave and sorry for myself. I didn't think much of the baby but of my own body and what it had just been through. What it might start to feel like in the hours and days to come. How I might survive.

And then he was brought into the room. The same baby who had been wedged inside me all these hours was now being presented to me swaddled in a pale blue hospital blanket with a hand-knitted mint-green hat. He weighed 8lb 6 ounces and was 58cm long. Here and there his hat was encrusted with patches of blood, already turning brown. His or mine, I do not know. Ours. He was placed on my chest, his little mouth working already at the smell of me. I craned my neck forward, unsure of how to hold him. His skin was dry and the top of his head smelt like biscuit dough. His eyes were closed. I made an effort to notice him more but I was so exhausted it was an act of will rather than desire. His skin was sallow, more pale than I expected. He had my big squashy nose, my father's nose, and a dainty rosebud mouth, the top lip slightly overhanging. I saw elegant long fingers. A serious expression. A life.

I said nothing, lay back stunned on the gurney. We were wheeled out of theatre to the recovery room. Claire walked behind us, her slow footsteps squeaking on the gleaming floors. The baby lay still, settled, and precious on my chest. I watched the panelled ceiling race away from us as we moved forward slowly, tenderly, ceremonially. A little life procession down a hospital corridor at the start of another day. A beginning, after all.

Select Bibliography

The Handmaid's Tale, Margaret Atwood, Virago, 1990

The Safety of the Unborn Child, Geoffrey Chamberlain, Penguin, 1969

The Awakening, Kate Chopin, Canongate, 2014

'The Laugh of the Medusa', Helene Cixous, University of Chicago Press, *Signs*, Vol. 1, No. 4 (Summer, 1976)

Newborn, Kate Clanchy, Picador, 2004

Maternity: Letters From Working Women, edited by Margaret Llewelyn Davies, Virago, 1978

Making Babies: Stumbling into Motherhood, Anne Enright, Vintage, 2005

Heartburn, Nora Ephron, Virago, 2008

Ina May's Guide to Childbirth, Ina May Gaskin, Vermilion, 2008

Jizzen, Kathleen Jamie, Picador, 1999

Ulysses, James Joyce, Penguin, 1992 (original edition, 1922)

The Birth of Love, Joanna Kavenna, Faber, 2010

The Namesake, Jhumpa Lahiri, Harper Perennial, 2004

Beloved, Toni Morrison, Vintage, 1997

The Virago Book Of Birth Poetry, edited by Charlotte Otten, Virago, 1993

Collected Poems, Sylvia Plath, Faber, 1981

The Journals of Sylvia Plath 1950–1962, Sylvia Plath, Faber, 2014

Bibliography

Winter Trees, Sylvia Plath, Faber, 2010 Kindle edition

Your Pregnancy Week By Week, Lesley Regan, professor of obstetrics and gynaecology, Dorling Kindersley, 2010 revised edition

Out Of Silence: selected poems, Muriel Rukeyser, edited by Kate Daniels, TriQuarterly Books/Northwestern University Press, 1994

The Rings of Saturn, WG Sebald, Vintage, 2002

Frankenstein, Mary Shelley, Everyman's Library, 1992 (original edition, 1818)

The Living Mountain, Nan Shepherd, Canongate, 2011 (original edition, 1977, written 1940s)

This Giving Birth: Pregnancy and Childbirth in American Women's Writing, edited by Julie Tharp and Susan MacCallum-Whitcomb, Bowling Green State University Popular Press, 2000

Anna Karenina, Leo Tolstoy, Penguin, 2006 (original full Russian edition, 1878)

Misconceptions, Naomi Wolf, Vintage, 2002

The Second Common Reader, Virginia Woolf, Pelican, 1944

A Room of One's Own, Virginia Woolf, Penguin, 1945 (original edition, 1929)

Acknowledgements

Thanks to all the people who made this book possible. Jenny Brown, my agent, who is just as wonderful as everyone says she is and who read the first few chapters, instructed me to keep going, and has been keeping me right ever since. Sara Hunt, my publisher, for her unwavering belief, and Ali Moore, the most enthusiastic of editors. I'm still waiting to hear the stories of the green beans, Auntie Agnes and the Reader's Digest photoshoot...

Thanks to Jennifer Smith and Jonathan Hope, who have supported this book from the outset in every way possible. Tracey Black, for being such a quietly encouraging early reader and for regularly looking after the boy born at the end of this book while I tried to write the damn thing. Stuart Kelly, Peggy Hughes and Claire Stewart: a formidable trio who give the most sound, stylish and well-oiled counsel.

Finally, my deepest thanks to my family, the ones who conceived me until I could conceive of myself. My wonderfully idiosyncratic parents, whom I interviewed for chapter six, producing one of the most fascinating, hilarious, moving and occasionally unreliable conversations of our relationship. My sister, for the nights spent listening to 'Tajabone'. My dog Daphne, for the warm fur, wise expressions and wordlessness. And deepest thanks to Claire, first reader, editor, partner, and now co-parent. This story belongs to her too.

Every effort has been made to contact the rights holders for permission to reproduce quotations and extracts from works referenced in this book; thanks are due to all of them.

Acknowledgements

Quotation from *The Handmaid's Tale*, © Margaret Atwood, published by Jonathan Cape. Reproduced by permission of The Random House Group Ltd.

Quotations from 'Laugh of the Medusa', © Hélène Cixous, transl. Keith Cohen and Paula Cohen, *Signs*, 1976, University of Chicago Press.

Extract from 'Thaw', © Kathleen Jamie, reprinted by kind permission of the author.

Quotation from *The Namesake*, © Jhumpa Lahiri, Harper Perennial (permission requested).

Quotation from *Beloved* by Toni Morrison, published by Chatto & Windus. Reproduced by permission of The Random House Group Ltd. From *Song of Solomon* by Toni Morrison, published by Chatto & Windus. Reproduced by permission of The Random House Group Ltd.

Excerpt from 'The Language of the Brag' from *Satan Says*, by Sharon Olds, ©1980. Reprinted by permission of the University of Pittsburgh Press.

Quotations from Sylvia Plath: 'Metaphors' from *Collected Poems*, *The Journals of Sylvia Plath* 1950–1962; *Winter Trees*, all published by, and reproduced by permission of, Faber & Faber and © Estate of Sylvia Plath.

The poem 'Islands' from *The Gates*, 1978 'Nine Poems for the Unborn Child' from *The Green Wave*, 1948: © Muriel Rukeyser, reprinted by kind permission of ICM, New York.

Quotations from Nan Shepherd, *The Living Mountain*, copyright © Nan Shepherd, 2008. First published in Great Britain in 1977 by Aberdeen University Press. Current editions published by Canongate Books Ltd.

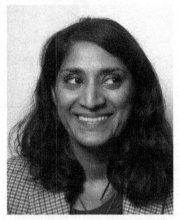

BOB MCDEVITT

Chitra Ramaswamy is an award-winning journalist. She cut her teeth at *The Big Issue in Scotland* before moving to *Scotland on Sunday* and later *The Scotsman*, where she became one of the newspaper's leading columnists, book reviewers, interviewers and feature writers. Now freelance, Chitra writes for *The Guardian* and a number of other publications and regularly appears on radio. She lives in Edinburgh with her partner, son and rescue dog. *Expecting* is her first book.